15,95

COLOR ATLAS OF
ORO-FACIAL DISEASES

YEAR BOOK *Color Atlas Series*
Series Editor
G. BARRY CARRUTHERS, M.D. (Lond.)

Color Atlas of General Pathology
Color Atlas of Ophthalmological Diagnosis
Color Atlas of Oro-Facial Diseases

Further titles now in preparation
Color Atlas of Histological & Cytological Techniques
Color Atlas of Gynecology
Color Atlas of Dermatology
Color Atlas of Pediatrics
Color Atlas of Infectious Diseases
Color Atlas of Venereology
Color Atlas of Bacteriology
Color Atlas of Renal Diseases
Color Atlas of Physical Signs in Clinical Medicine
Color Atlas of Tropical Medicine
Color Atlas of Parasitology
Color Atlas of Forensic Medicine
Color Atlas of Orthopedics
Color Atlas of the Liver
Color Atlas of E.N.T. Diagnosis
Color Atlas of Virology
Color Atlas of Dental Surgery
Color Atlas of Cardiology
Color Atlas of Respiratory Diseases
Color Atlas of Endocrinology
Color Atlas of Surgical Diagnosis

COLOR ATLAS
OF
Oro-Facial Diseases

L. W. KAY
M.D.S., F.D.S., R.C.S., F.I.C.S., M.R.C.S. Eng., L.R.C.P. Lond.

Reader in Oral Surgery, University of London,
Consultant, Eastman Dental Hospital, London

and

R. HASKELL
M.B., B.S., B.D.S., M.R.C.P., F.D.S., R.C.S.

Consultant Dental Surgeon,
King's College Hospital, London

YEAR BOOK MEDICAL PUBLISHERS, INC.
35 E. WACKER DRIVE–CHICAGO

© L. W. Kay & R. Haskell, 1971

This book is copyrighted in England and may not be reproduced by any means in whole or in part.

Distributed in Continental North, South, and Central America, Hawaii, Puerto Rico, and the Philippines by

YEAR BOOK MEDICAL PUBLISHERS, INC.

by arrangement with

WOLFE PUBLISHING LIMITED

Library of Congress Catalog Card Number: 79-153-288
International Standard Book Number: 0-8151-5000-8

Printed by Smeets-Weert Holland

Acknowledgements

It is with great pleasure that we record our gratitude to Mr. W. J. Morgan of the Photographic Department at the Institute of Dental Surgery of the University of London for his skilled technical assistance and authoritative advice. We are also indebted to Mrs. B. Rayiru for her untiring secretarial help. In preparing a volume such as this, the compilers inevitably have to rely upon the generosity of colleagues who are able to supply a copy of "the picture that got away" or the lesion which never did pass through our clinic. It is, therefore, with great appreciation that we acknowledge the assistance of the following benefactors – Professor H. C. Killey, Mr. N. L. Rowe, Professor G. B. Winter, Mr. J. D. Manson, Mr. F. G. Hardman, Mr. J. H. Sowray, Dr. F. F. Nally, Mr. R. Brooks, Dr. J. C. Southam, Mr. P. H. Morse, Mr. R. C. W. Dinsdale and Mr. B. Williams. We are most grateful also to Messrs. E. & S. Livingstone of Edinburgh for permission to reproduce Fig. 36, and to Messrs. John Wright & Sons of Bristol for permission to reproduce Fig. 137.

L. W. KAY
R. HASKELL
1971

Contents

Introduction 8

SECTION ONE
   Face and Neck 10

SECTION TWO
   The Abscess 42

SECTION THREE
   The Teeth 64

SECTION FOUR
   The Gingivae 102

SECTION FIVE
   The "Lumps" 126

SECTION SIX
   Prosthetic Problems 166

SECTION SEVEN
   The Palate 172

SECTION EIGHT
   The Tongue 188

SECTION NINE
   Radiopacities and Radiolucencies 196

SECTION TEN
   White Patches and Ulcers 222

SECTION ELEVEN
   Jaw Deformities 260

   Index 285

Introduction

THIS ATLAS provides a concise and representative record of many of the morphological variations and disease processes encountered in the clinical examination of the oro-facial region. Although designed primarily for medical and dental practitioners, the content of the book constitutes an instructive manual both for those undergoing clinical training as undergraduates and for those engaged in postgraduate study in the allied fields of oral diagnosis, medicine and surgery. It is also hoped that even the most experienced and perceptive members of the professions will find the collection of illustrations a useful diagnostic aide-memoire and a refresher course on the more obscure disease entities. Although a guide to intelligent diagnosis, a book of this type must never be regarded as a substitute for the detailed practical study of actual cases.

A simple but logical plan has been adopted in setting out the material in this work. The contents are arranged in sections, on a clinico-anatomical basis, each of which covers a group of distinct lesions showing points of resemblance to each other. It is thus possible to emphasise important distinguishing clinical features.

Although a classification either on an aetiological or pathological basis has been dispensed with, the authors would like to stress that in the assembly of the illustrations the format chosen is not intended to be an endorsement of spot diagnosis but rather to underline the value of a full and careful case history supported by a complete clinical examination. Where appropriate, both clinical and radiological photographs of the lesion are shown. Obviously, as the saying goes, a good picture is worth a thousand words, especially if complemented by an apt and succinct descriptive caption. The space allotted to the legends has been necessarily restricted to a few lines, but this permits the resourceful reader an opportunity to amplify the short text with personal notes on the respective subject matter. Those who require more factual information should consult the standard textbooks and pertinent monographs.

In order to achieve a uniform classification and terminology for the diseases cited, the nomenclature has been based on the International Classification of Diseases (ICD-DA) published by the World Health Organisation in 1969; and the appropriate code numbers are provided for the purpose of easy identification.

SECTION ONE: **FACE and NECK**

Fig. 1. The typical facies in mitral stenosis. Such patients require antibiotic prophylaxis for oral surgery procedures as do all patients with a history of congenital and acquired cardiac defects with disturbed blood flow.

Fig. 2. The facies of congenital "specific disease" with a collapsed nasal bridge. Hutchinson's incisors, perceptive deafness and interstitial keratitis are associated features. *(090-5)*

Fig. 3. Herpes zoster affecting the second and third divisions of the trigeminal nerve of a patient with von Recklinghausen's neurofibromatosis. The neurofibromas are soft and most are cutaneous. Zoster is characterised by pre-eruption pain followed by a chicken-pox rash in the distribution of the affected nerve. *(053.XO; 743.40)*

Fig. 4. Paget's disease of bone affecting the skull, maxilla and right zygoma. Note the enlarged calvarium and right facial bones. Paget's disease of the skull bones is usually painless and is noted as an incidental finding. *(721.XO)*

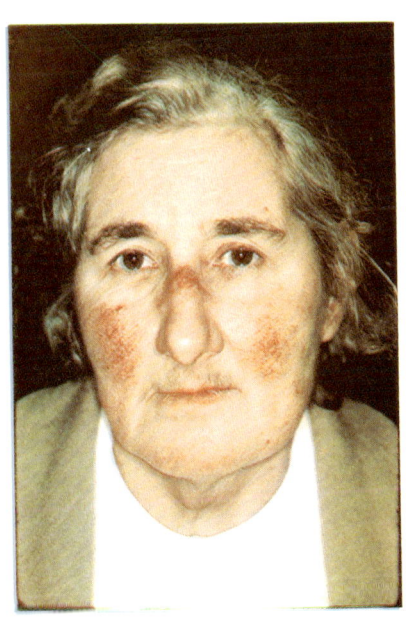
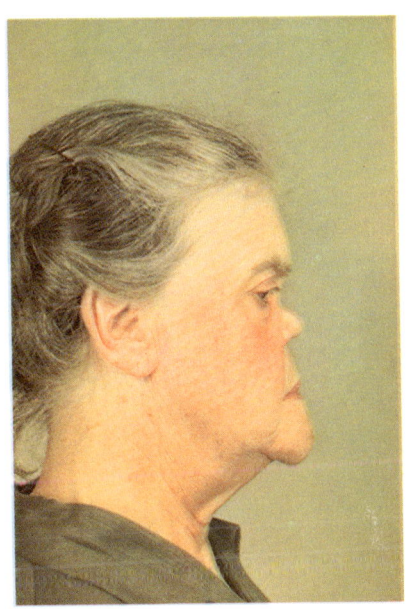
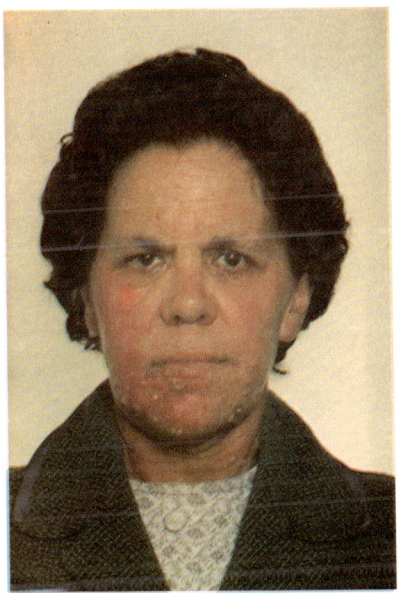
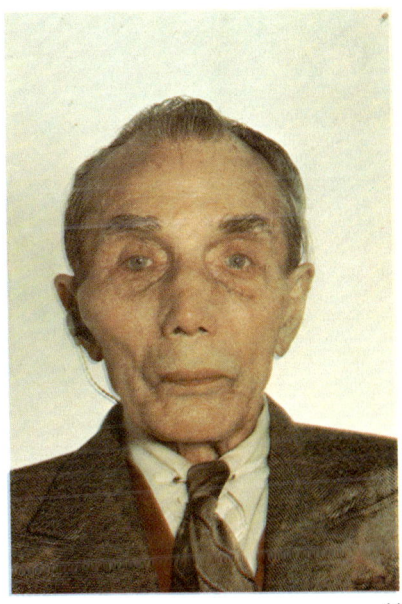

Fig. 5. A facial rash due to penicillin allergy. Caution is essential before penicillin is given, the patient being questioned by both the prescriber and the nurse giving an injection of the drug. *(N960)*

Fig. 6. A scarlatiniform rash affecting the whole body, again due to penicillin hypersensitivity. Severe and even fatal reactions may occur from this cause, but a rash such as this is appropriately treated by withdrawing the drug, prescribing an antihistamine and warning the patient against future exposure to any of the penicillins. *(N960)*

Fig. 7. Angioneurotic oedema of the lower lip. Such recurrent swellings of the face may be wrongly attributed to dental infection. Characteristically the swelling develops rapidly and painlessly and remits within a few hours. Occasionally an allergen can be identified. *(708.00)*

Fig. 8. Bleeding into the tissues of the face in a patient on anticoagulant therapy. Clinically in such cases the swelling can bear a close resemblance to a dental abscess and a misguided extraction might prove hazardous. *(N964)*

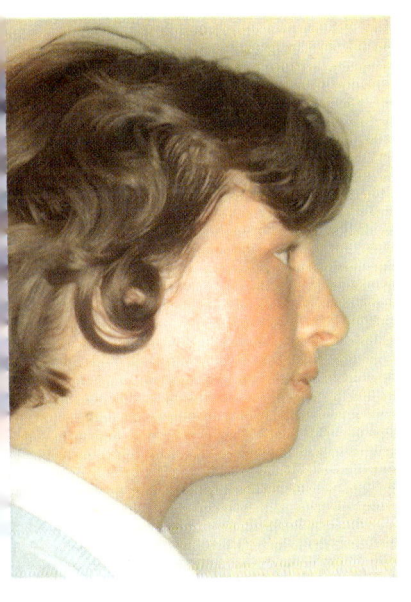
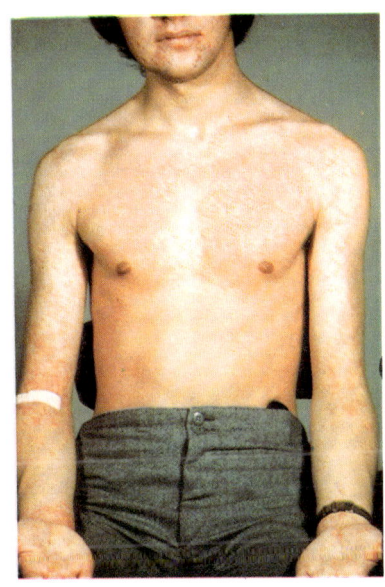
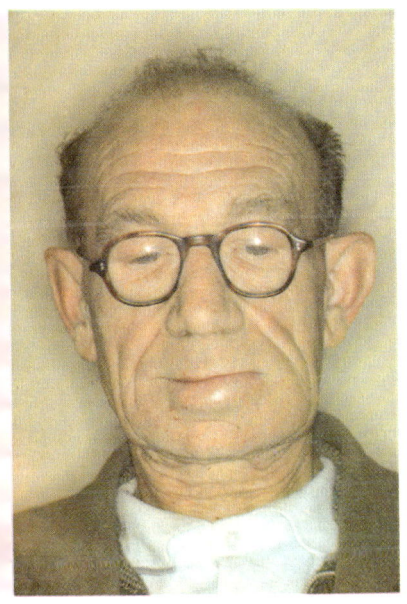
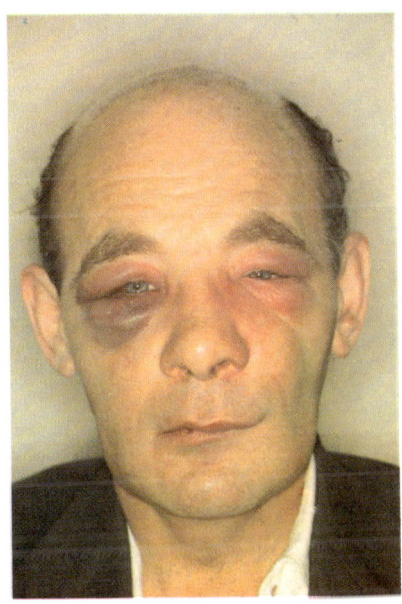

13

Fig. 9. Surgical emphysema of the face which may complicate dental treatment. Again, the resemblance to an acute infection is striking, but it is only superficial. The swelling occurs suddenly following various forms of dental treatment or trauma, and is soft. Crepitus is not always elicitable. *(N997)*

Fig. 10. Facial palsy, in this case as a hallmark of the Ramsey-Hunt syndrome in which herpes zoster affects the seventh cranial nerve. Pain occurs in the ear, followed by vesiculation there and also sometimes on the soft palate. *(053.X0)*

Fig. 11. Oxycephaly, showing the deformed cranium and the "copper-beaten" skull. *(756.05)*

Fig. 12. Clinical picture of the patient. This is one variety of the craniostenoses in which premature closure of sutures leads to deformation of the skull.

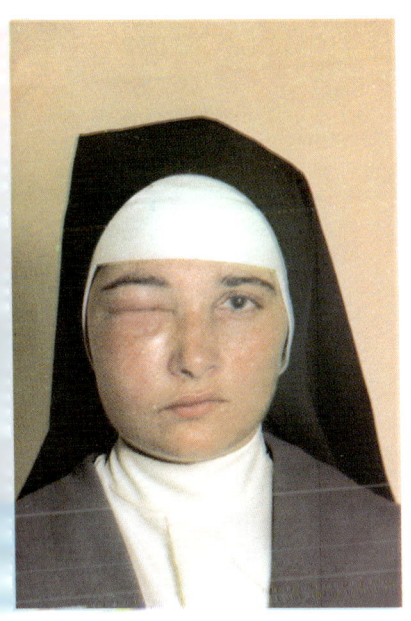
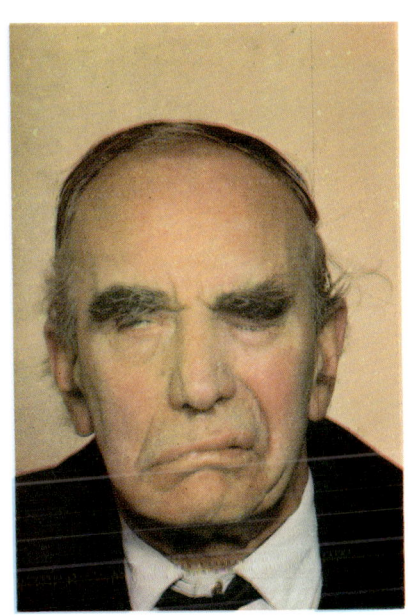
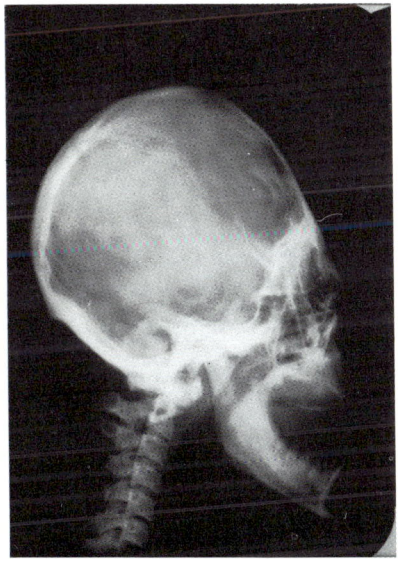
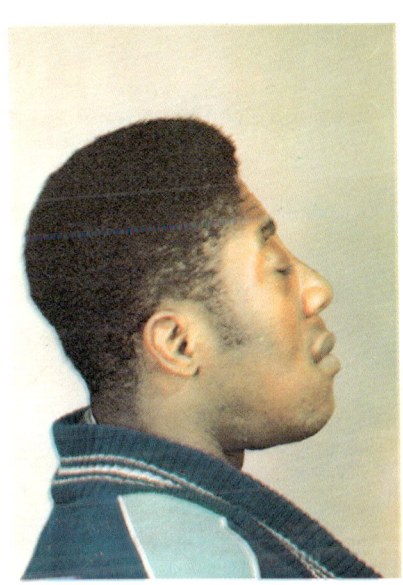

Fig. 13. The maxillary alveolus much expanded by Paget's disease (the same case as **fig. 4**). Following tooth extraction on the right side, sequestration occurred. This is a common complication of this bone dystrophy, and it is fortunate that Paget's disease does not affect the mandible. The typical alteration in the plasma is a rise in the alkaline phosphatase; the calcium and phosphorus levels remain normal. *(721.X0)*

Fig. 14. An x-ray of the same case shows the fluffy bone production typical of Paget's disease with great thickening of the skull.

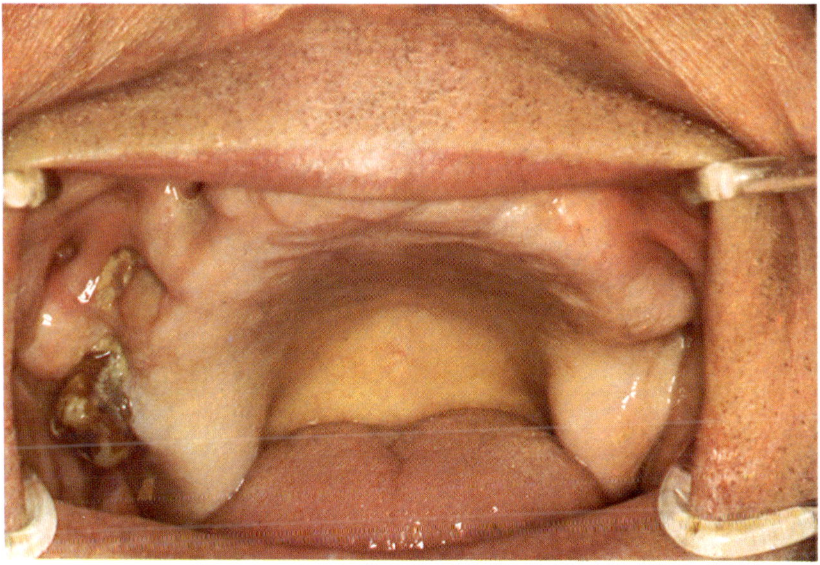

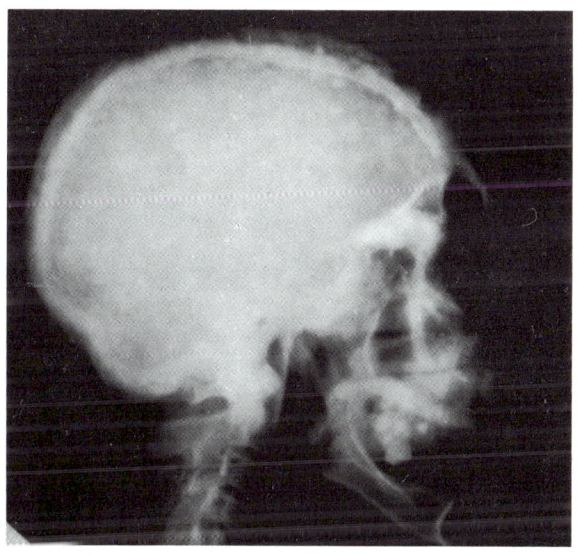

Figs. 15 & 16. This boy has a soft swelling of the right cheek which has been enlarging since birth. The intra-oral view shows the lesion with a pebbly surface. It is a lymphangioma. *(227.X0)*

Figs. 17 & 18. Capillary haemangioma of the face accompanied by an ipsilateral angioma of the cerebral hemisphere (which later calcifies). The patient also has a haemangioma of the hand. This combination of signs is referred to as the Sturge-Weber syndrome. *(759.80)*

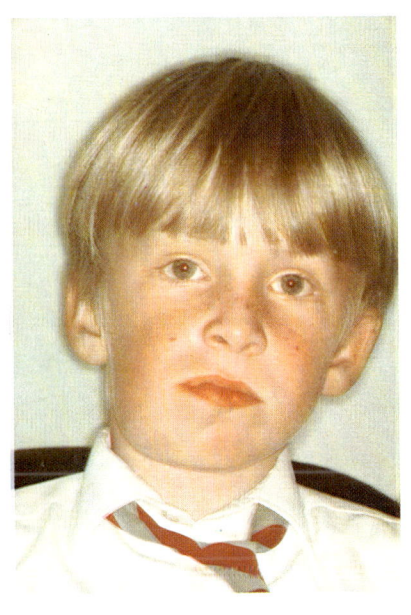
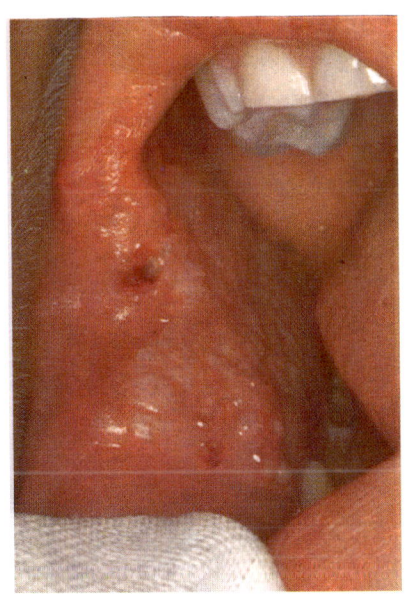
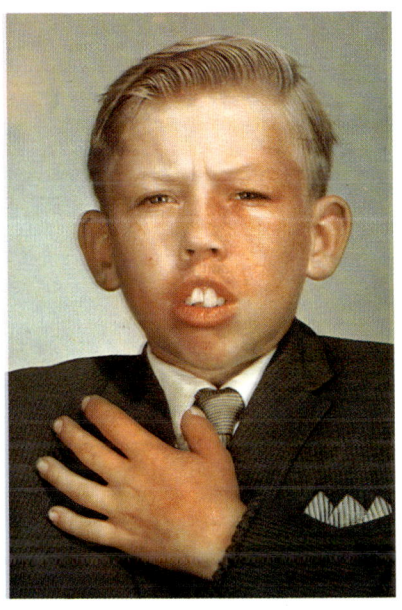
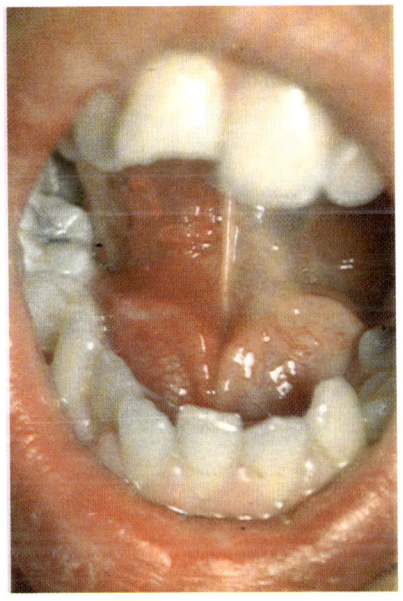

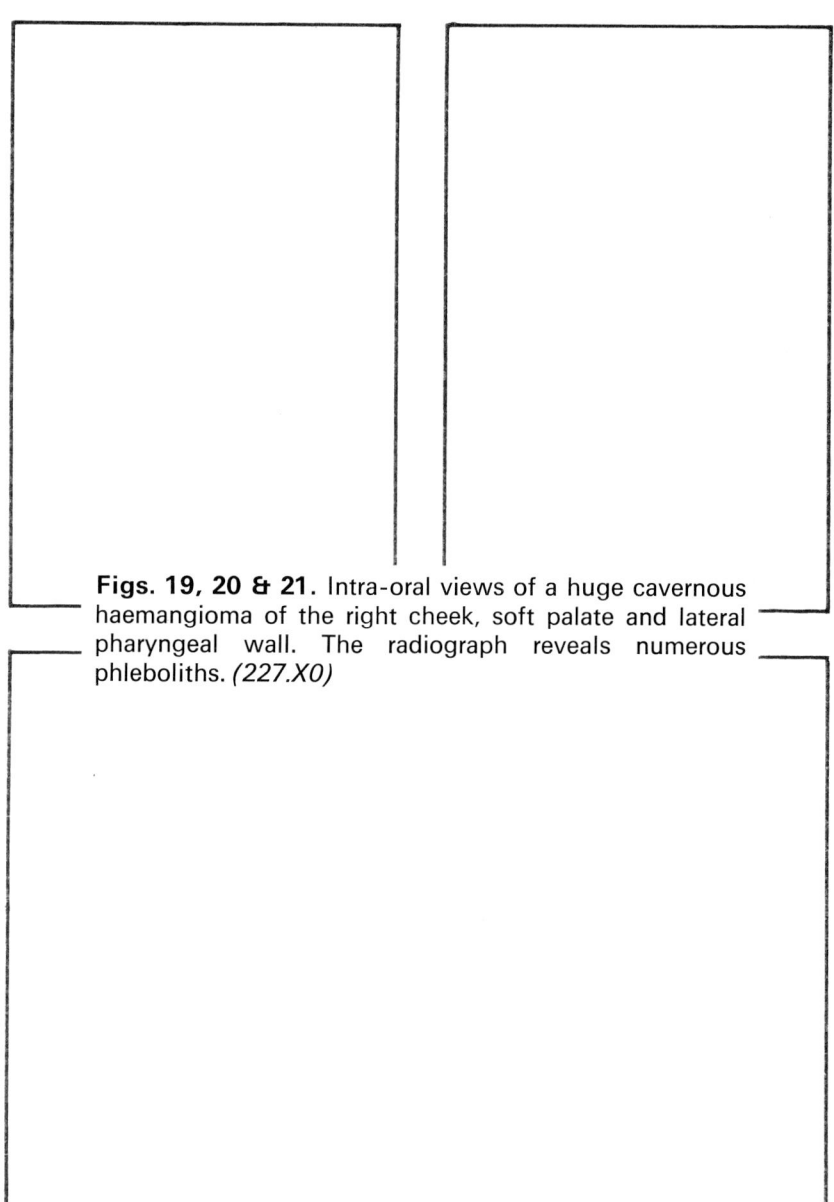

Figs. 19, 20 & 21. Intra-oral views of a huge cavernous haemangioma of the right cheek, soft palate and lateral pharyngeal wall. The radiograph reveals numerous phleboliths. *(227.X0)*

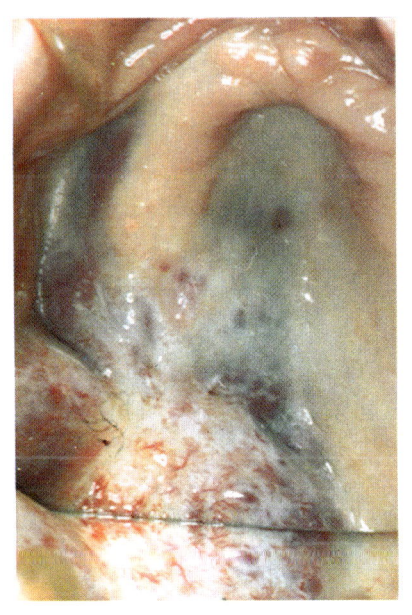
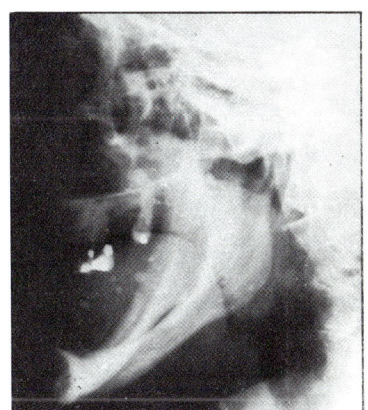

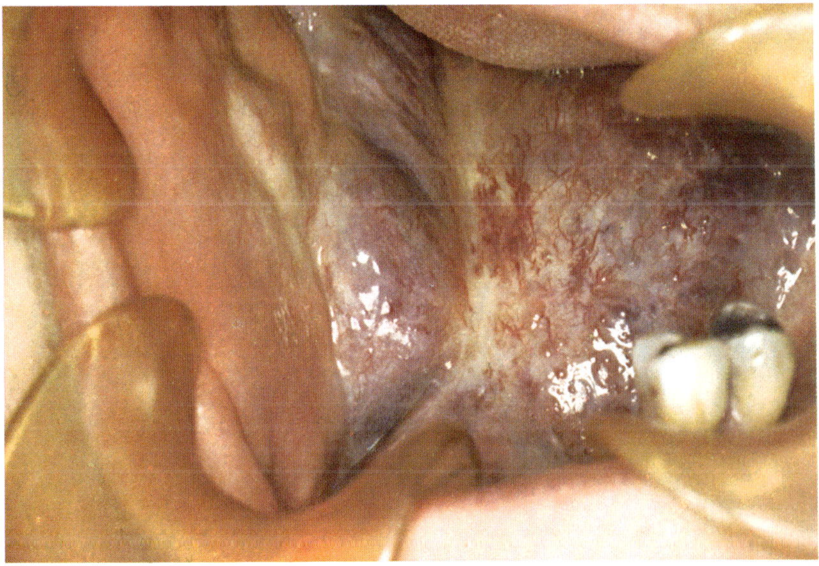

Fig. 22. This inconspicuous lesion on the side of the nose is a basal cell carcinoma. Note the slightly raised nodular edge with a white pearly cast. It is not yet ulcerated. *(173.3X)*

Fig. 23. A nodular plaque of lupus vulgaris (dermal tuberculosis). There is dusky erythema with many small papules which are, in fact, tubercles. The lesion enlarges slowly, destroying tissue with much scarring. *(017.0)*

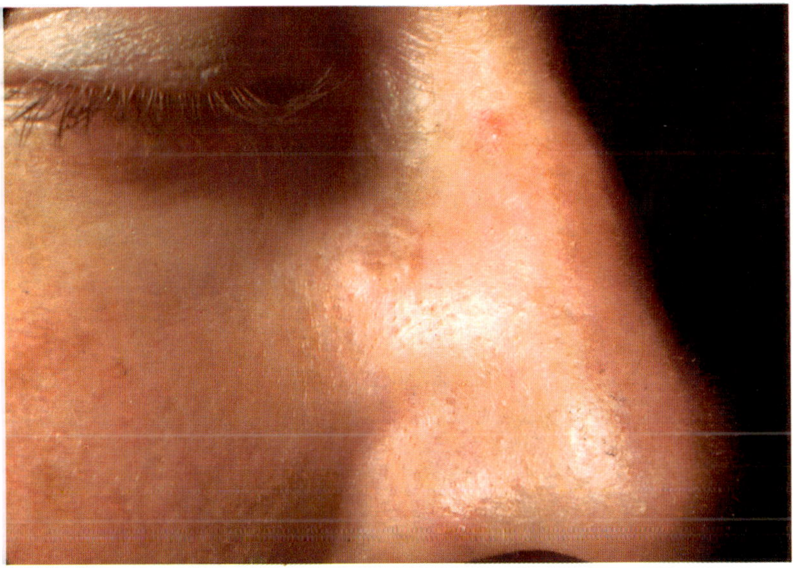

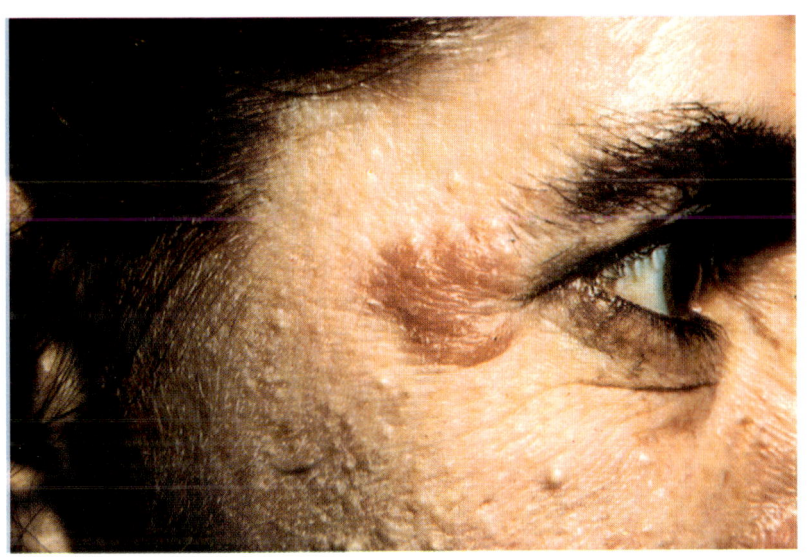

23

Fig. 24. A sebaceous cyst of the cheek with keratinised material exuding from the centre (a giant comedone).

Fig. 25. Malignant melanoma of the cheek. This shiny black lesion is slightly raised, rapidly enlarging, and associated with regional lymphadenopathy. *(172.3X)*

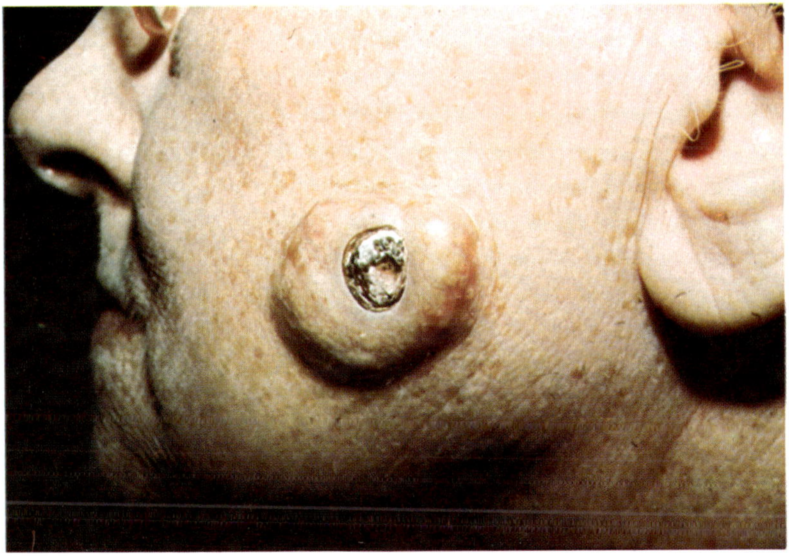

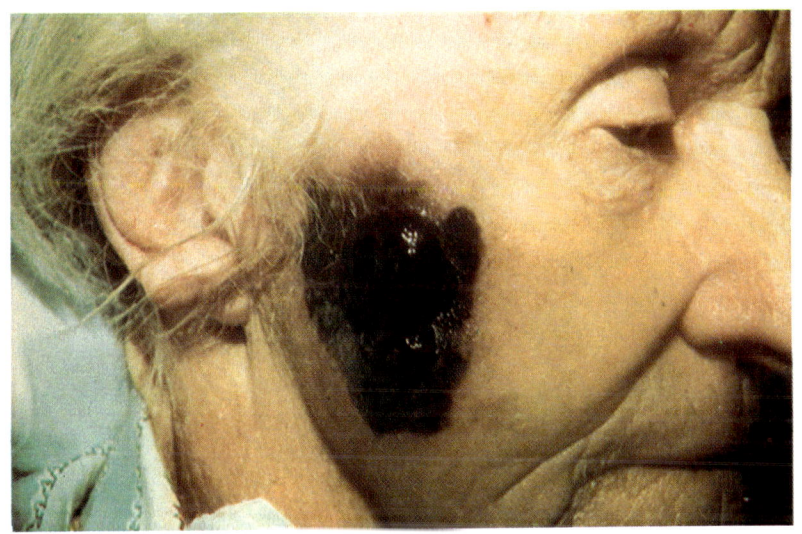

Fig. 26. The same case as **fig. 3.** The lesions of neurofibromatosis are well seen. *(053.X0; 743.40)*

Fig. 27. A pleomorphic adenoma of the parotid gland with a typically nodular surface. Such adenomas are slow-growing but may reach a large size. *(210.20)*

Fig. 28. The blue sclera seen in osteogenesis imperfecta. The colour is due to the pigmented choroid showing through the sclera, hypoplastic as a result of the mesenchymal defect. *(756.50)*

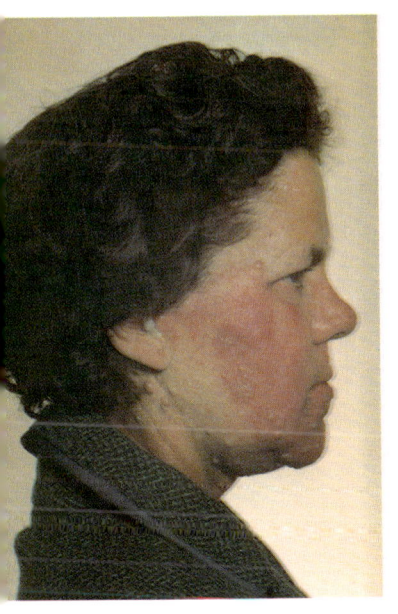
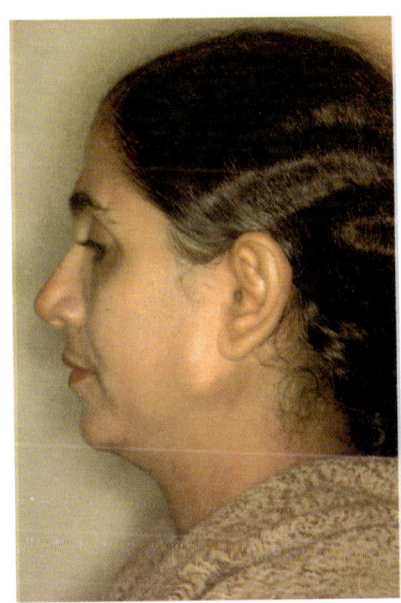

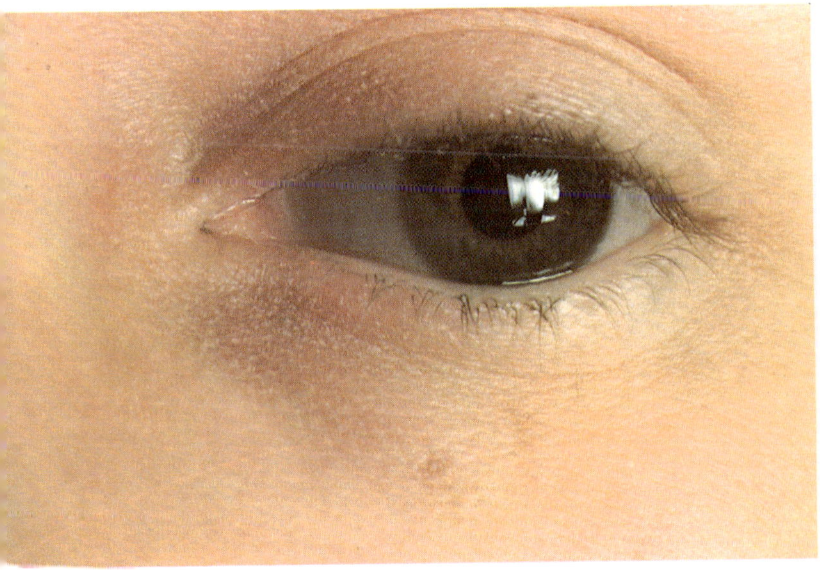

Fig. 29. Ecchymosis of the lip (and a herpetic lesion) in a pale, ill woman—a presentation of acute leukaemia which may be accompanied by symptoms of bleeding, infection or anaemia. *(207.V0)*

Fig. 30. Typical cavernous "haemangioma" of the lip. The swelling is completely compressible and such a lesion is common on the lips of the elderly. It is probably a varicosity rather than a haemangioma. *(227.X0)*

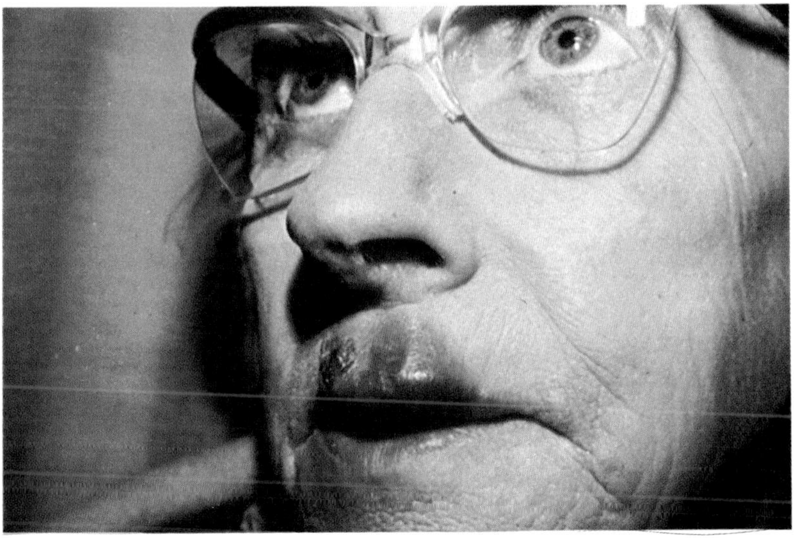

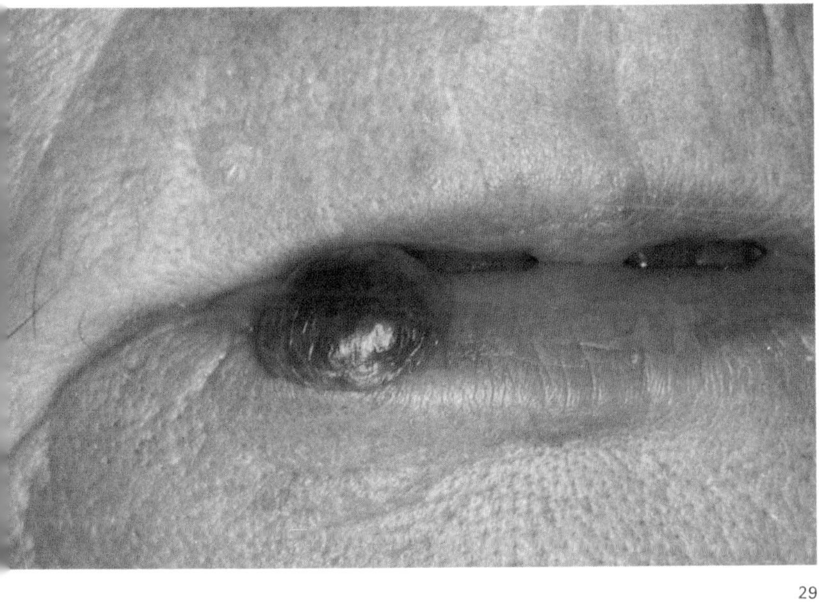

29

Fig. 31. Extensive actinic hyperkeratosis of the lower lip. Such epithelium is frequently dyskeratotic and is precancerous. *(528.58)*

Fig. 32. Multiple lesions of herpes labialis; these vesicles will rapidly break down and crust over. *(054.X0)*

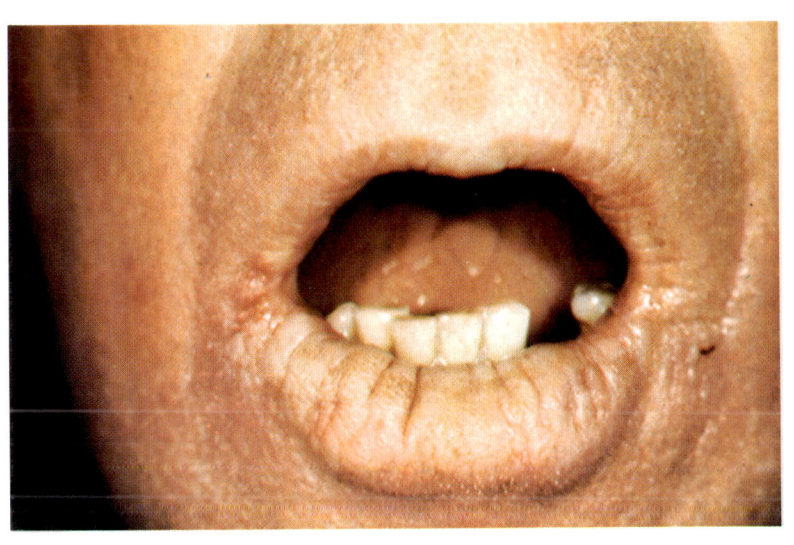

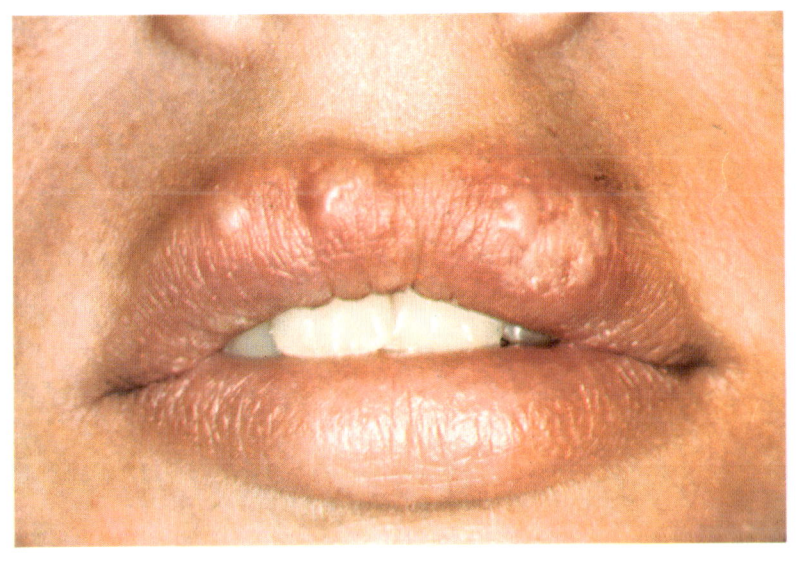

Fig. 33. Keratoacanthoma of the lower lip. A rapidly developing and spontaneously resolving lesion which closely resembles a squamous cell carcinoma — even histologically. *(210.03)*

Fig. 34. A squamous cell carcinoma of the lip which is a common neoplasm with a high five year cure-rate. *(140.10)*

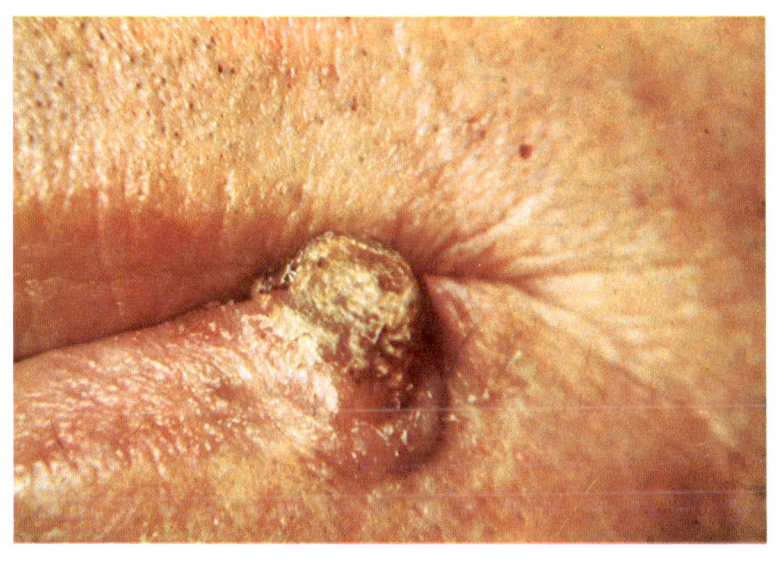

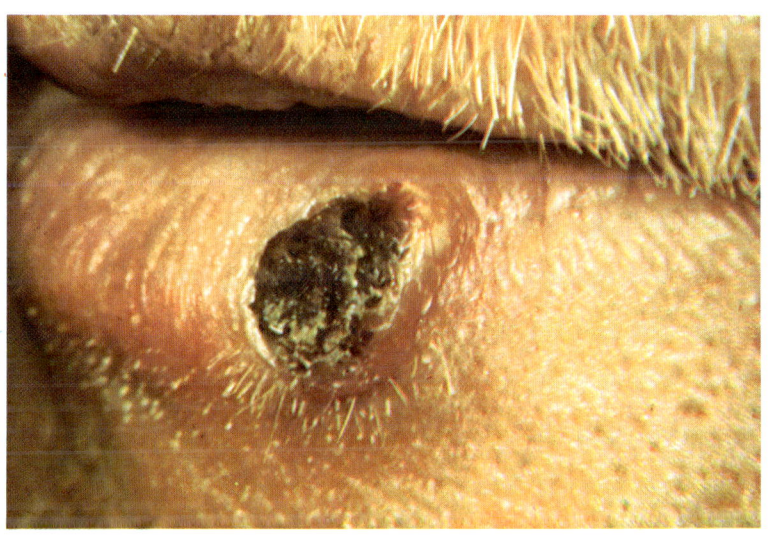

Fig. 35. A tiny papilloma of the lip commissure. Most oral papillomata are small. *(210.41)*

Fig. 36. A burn of the lips produced by inadequately cooled forceps during the extraction of teeth under general anaesthesia. *(998.99)*

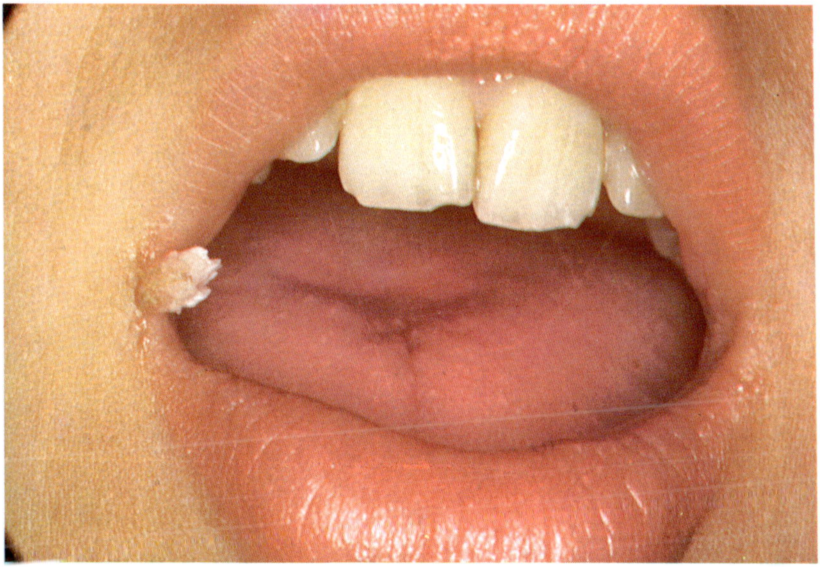

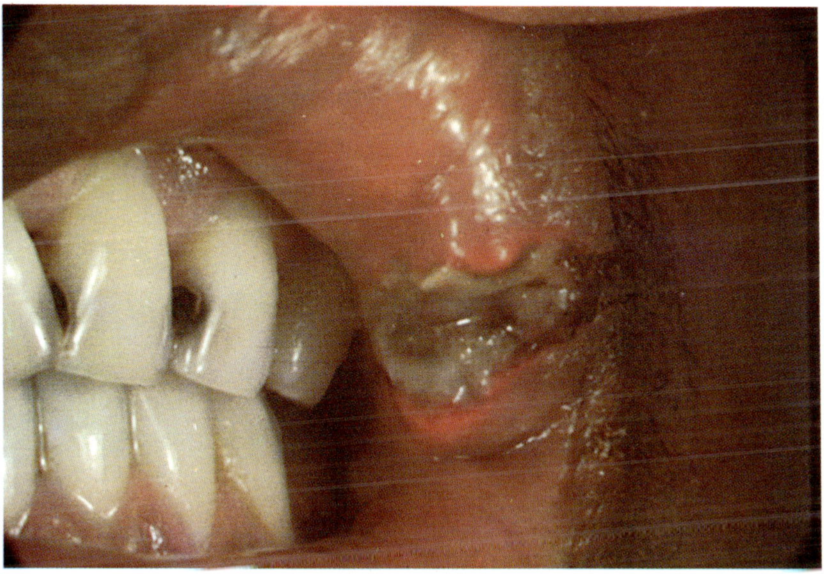

35

Fig. 37. The lips in the Peutz-Jegher's syndrome of gastro-intestinal (hamartomatous) polyposis with oral and digital pigmentation. The syndrome is characterised by gastro-intestinal bleeding, intermittent obstruction and only rarely by subsequent malignancy. The association with characteristic pigmentation makes a pre-operative diagnosis possible. *(750.90)*

Fig. 38. Hereditary haemorrhagic telangectasia showing the typical lesions. These are scattered through the nose and upper gastro-intestinal tract and bleeding may be occult, or overt from the nose and mouth. Obscure neurological episodes occur, dependent upon pulmonary arterio-venous aneurysms, which are also a feature. *(750.90)*

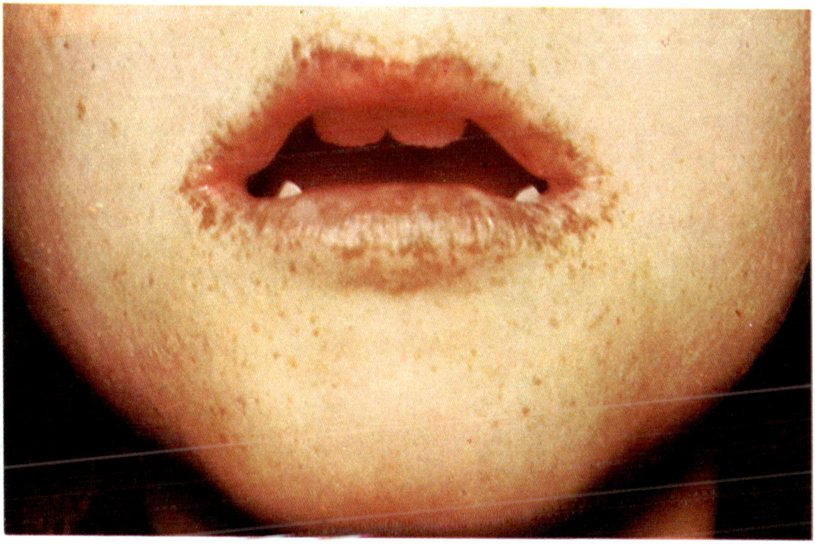

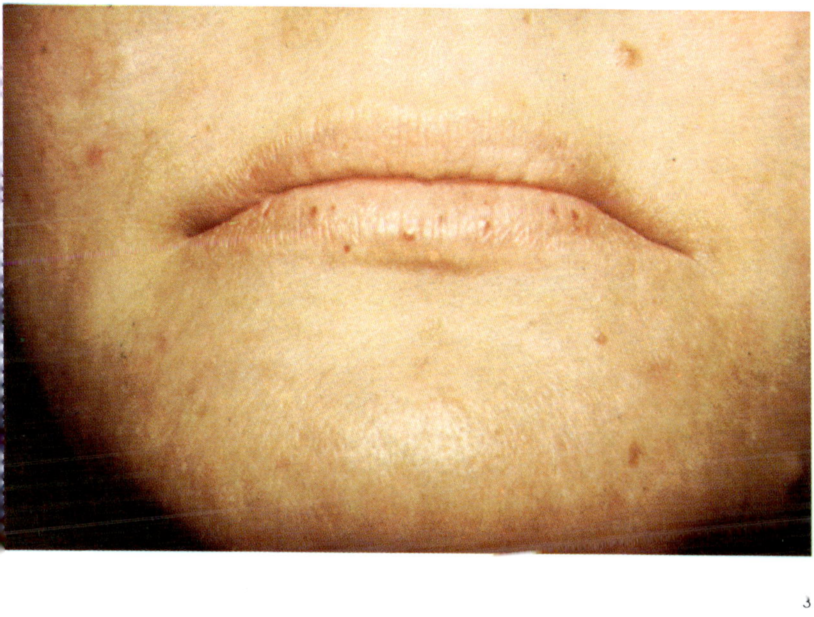

Fig. 39. A carbuncle of the chin. This is a skin infection usually due to staphylococci, but a dental abscess would have to be excluded in making the diagnosis. *(682.0X)*

Fig. 40. Extreme submandibular and sublingual swelling due to bleeding in the floor of the mouth in a patient on anticoagulants. The resemblance to an acute infection of these spaces is striking. *(N964)*

Fig. 41. Cancrum oris of the upper lip. This disease is a great rarity now in Europe but is not uncommon in African children. The proximate cause is a fuso-spirochaetal infection, but predisposing factors are of overwhelming importance. This condition is more likely to occur in the cheek. *(528.1X)*

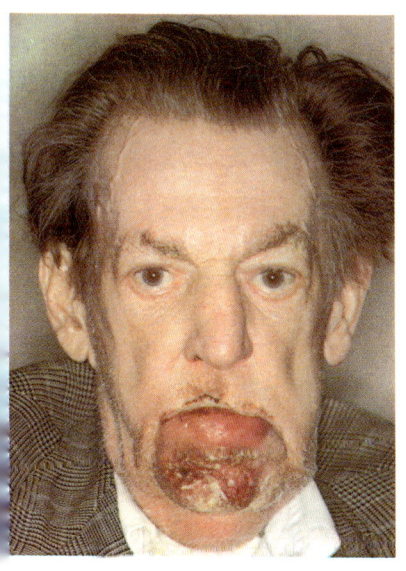
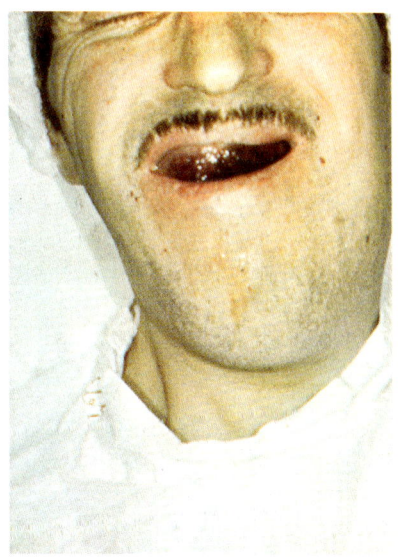
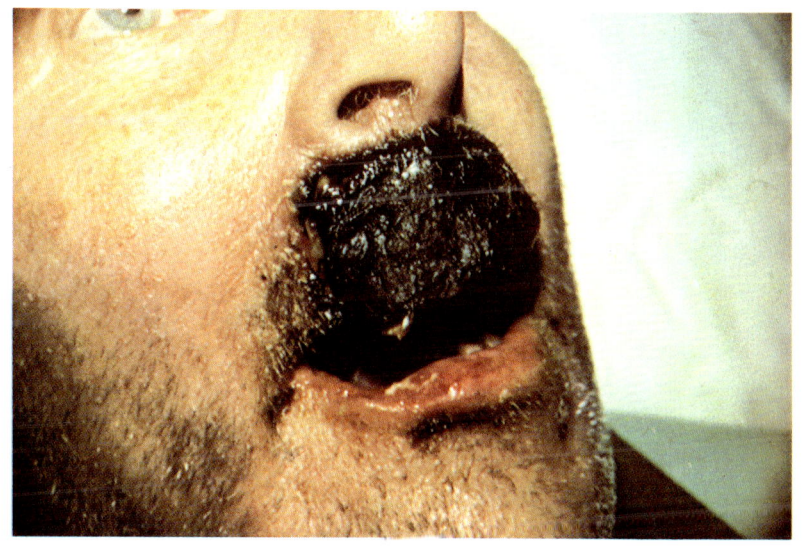

Fig. 42. Enlargement of the submandibular lymph nodes. This is a corollary of many dental infections; it may be quite marked with a minimal primary focus of infection and be the presenting feature, as here. *(683.X0)*

Fig. 43. Enlargement of the submandibular salivary gland due to obstruction of the duct by a stone. Characteristically in such a case the enlargement is post-prandial and painful, but eventually it also persists between meals. *(527.5X)*

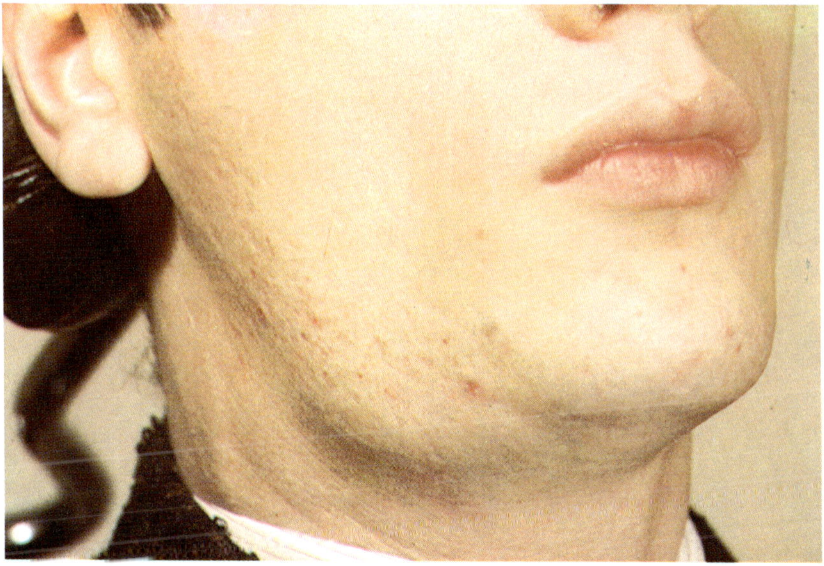

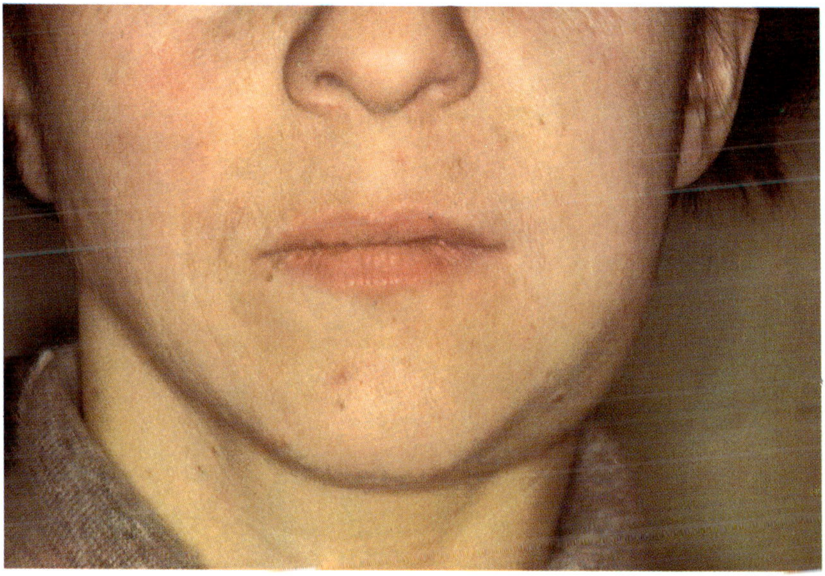

41

SECTION TWO: THE ABSCESS

Fig. 44. An acute dental abscess—here of the upper right first molar. The facial swelling is simply oedema—it is frequently misnamed cellulitis. *(522.5X)*

Fig. 45. This patient has extensive infection of the sublingual spaces and the right submandibular space. The infection followed extraction of the lower right second molar. *(528.3X)*

Figs. 46 & 47. A dental abscess presenting on the point of the chin. It has arisen from periodontal infection around the lower incisors, although the usual source is periapical infection of these teeth. If left untreated, the abscess will discharge to form a median mental sinus. The x-ray film reveals the extensive loss of alveolar bone due to the parodontal disease. *(522.5X)*

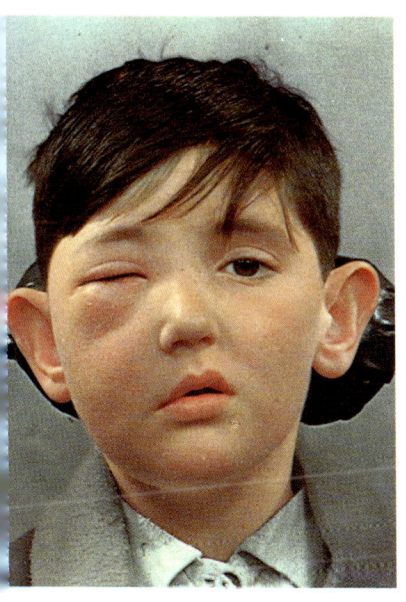
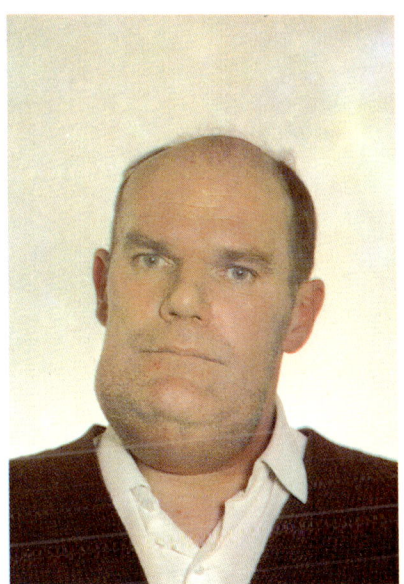
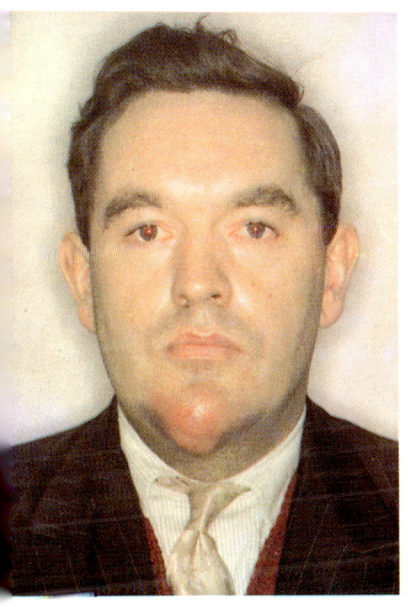
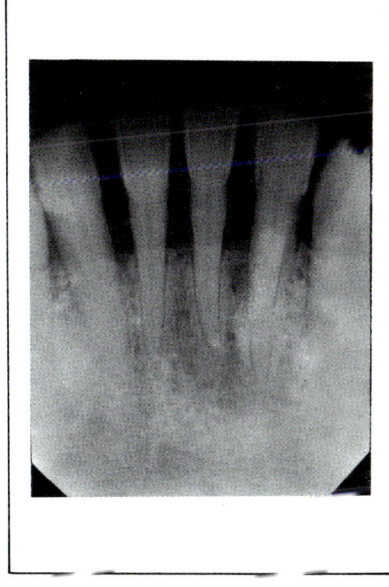

Fig. 48. Subacute actinomycosis with an abscess derived from the upper left first molar pointing on the face. Although sometimes initially an acute and severe infection, actinomycosis is marked by its persistence and a tendency to erode the adjacent skin. Diagnosis is established by bacteriological examination of pus obtained by aspiration. *(113.X0)*

Fig. 49. A dental infection (dento-alveolar abscess) pursuing an unusual course to discharge upon the face. At any sign of cutaneous involvement the abscess should be incised in order to prevent skin destruction and subsequent cicatrization. *(522.5X)*

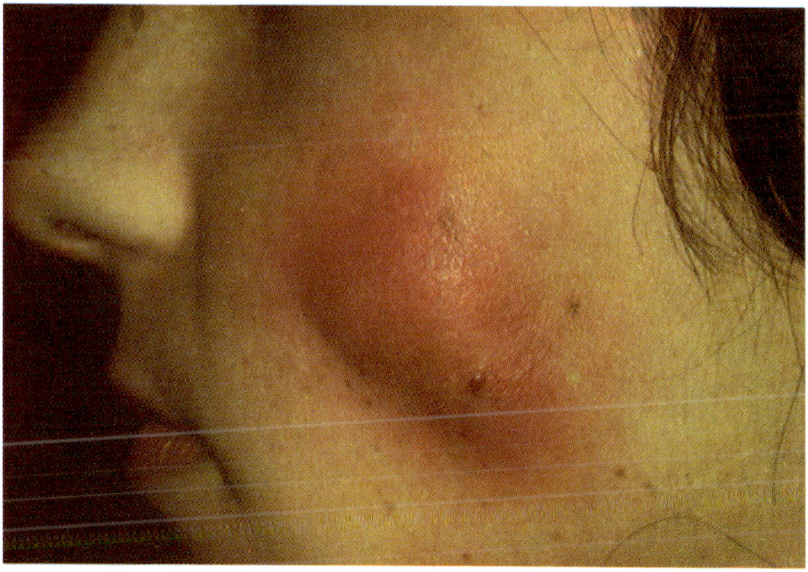

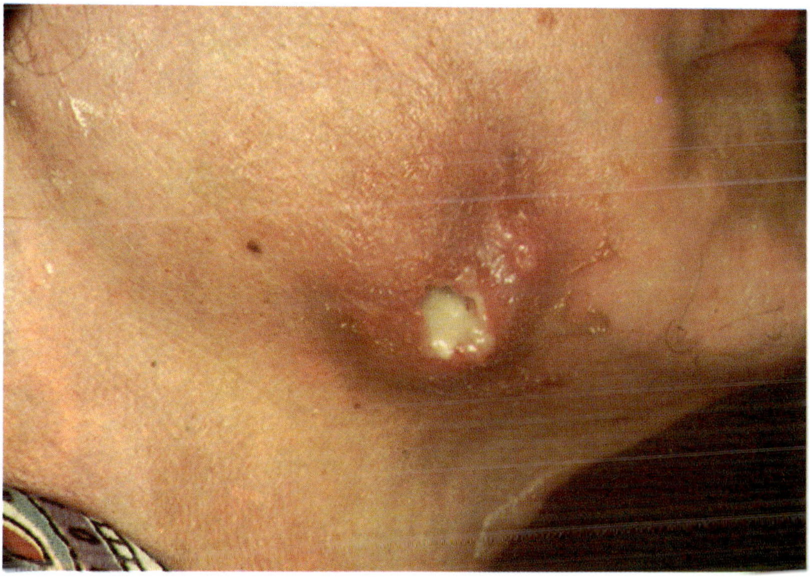

45

Fig. 50. An acute dental abscess presenting in the usual site — the labial or buccal sulcus. The tender swelling is clearly associated with the underlying bone and the overlying muscosa is inflamed. *(522.5X)*

Fig. 51. Another abscess, but here presenting in the lingual sulcus. The pus is subperiosteal — deep enough to give a bluish tint to the swelling. Such a swelling requires incision as well as removal of the offending tooth. *(522.5X)*

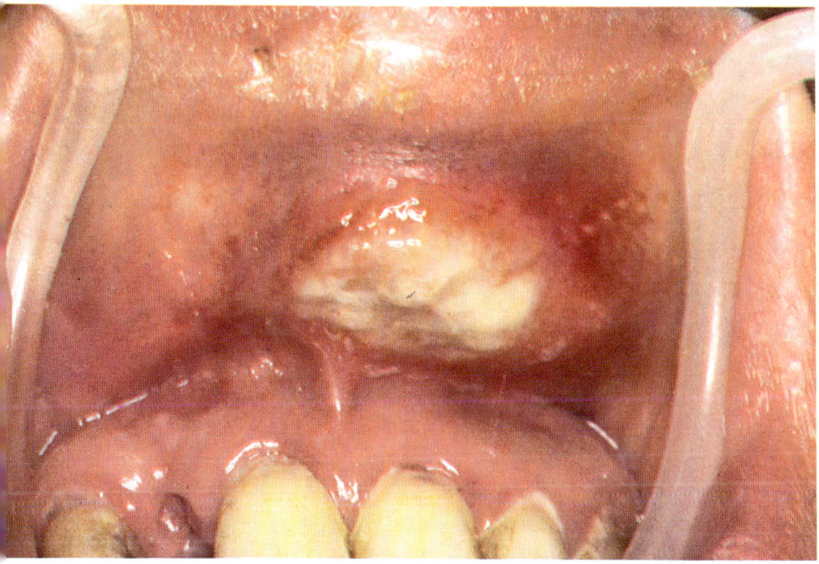

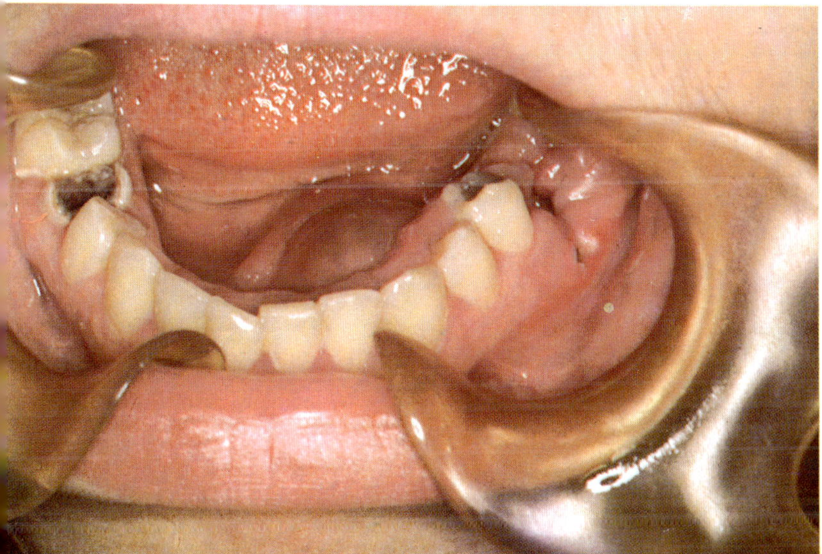

47

Fig. 52. A dental abscess derived from the roots of the right mandibular first molar which has discharged up the periodontal membrane. The mouth of the resulting sinus is surrounded by proliferative granulations which superficially resemble a pyogenic granuloma. *(522.5X)*

Fig. 53. Subacute abscess presenting on the face having tracked forward from a lower wisdom tooth subject to pericoronitis. *(523.42)*

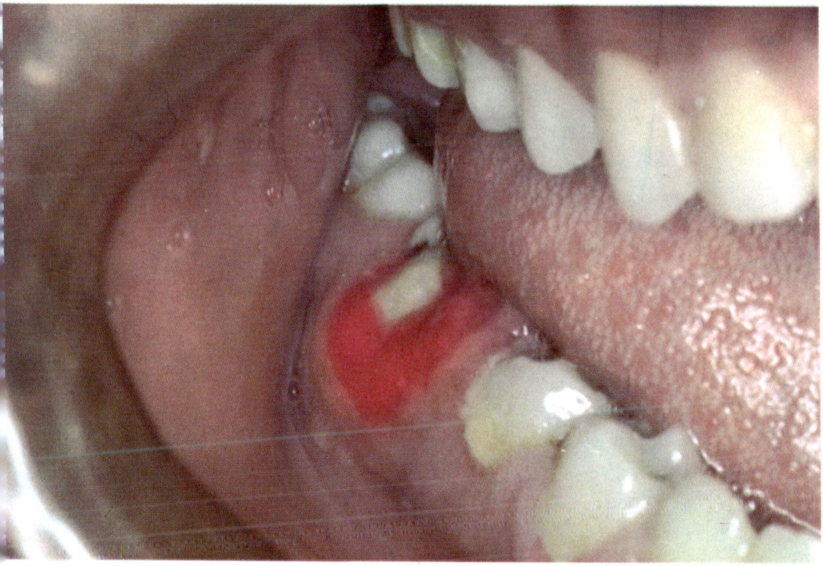

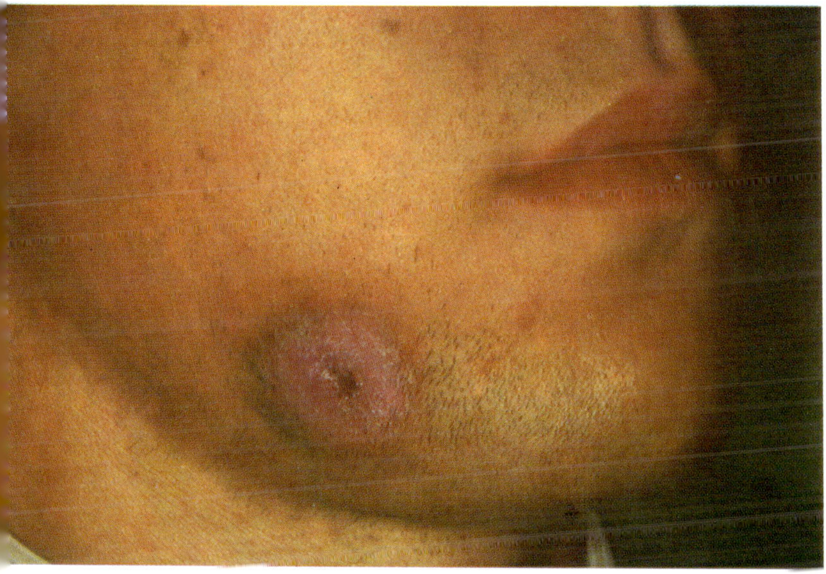

Fig. 54. Subacute pericoronitis; here, unusually, bilateral. In such cases the predisposing factor may be an upper respiratory tract infection or even infectious mononucleosis. *(523.42)*

Fig. 55. A migratory abscess resulting from acute pericoronitis associated with a third molar. Pus has tracked along the buccal sulcus to point opposite the lower first molar, which, unfortunately, is often removed abortively for relief of the symptoms. *(523.42)*

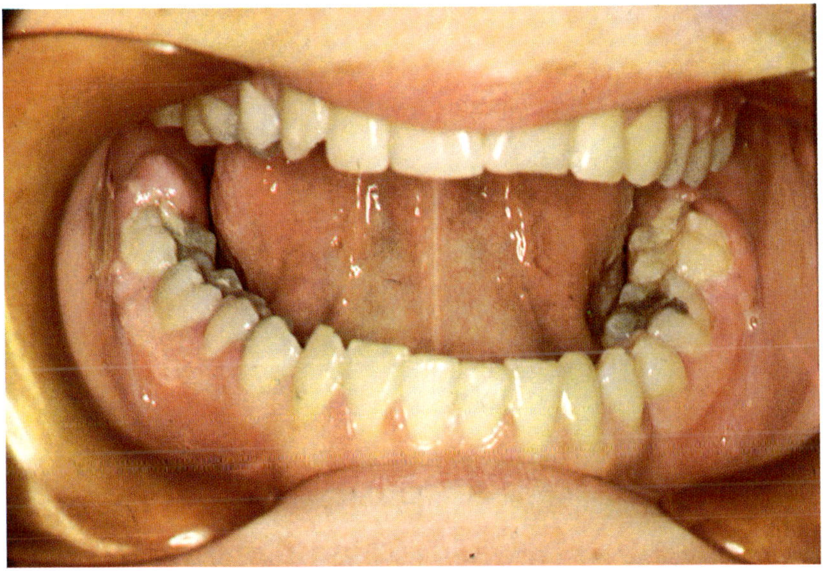

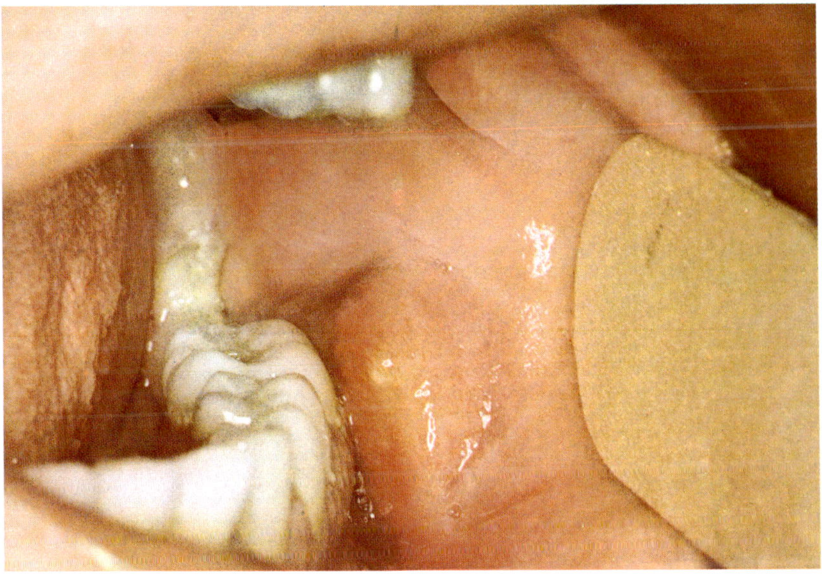

51

Fig. 56. Left facial swelling in the pre-auricular region due to a submasseteric abscess which can be a complication of pericoronitis or operative treatment of wisdom teeth. The pus strips up the periosteum and new bone is formed over the ascending ramus as in this x-ray view: **(Fig. 57)**. *(528.3X)*

Fig. 58. Again a submasseteric abscess, but here the cortical plate of the ascending ramus has sequestrated; this is one variety of subperiosteal osteomyelitis. Sequestration has occurred due to interruption of the periosteal blood supply, and the elevated periosteum has produced little new bone. Compare this with **fig. 57** in which the cortical plate has remained viable, and exuberant new bone formation has occurred. This disparity is largely attributable to the age of the patient and to a lesser extent to the nature of the underlying infection. *(528.3X)*

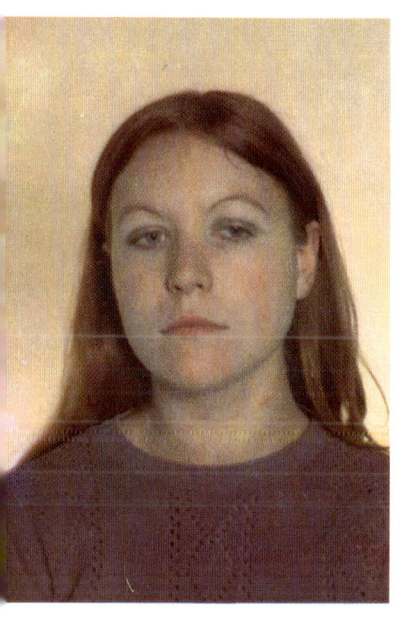
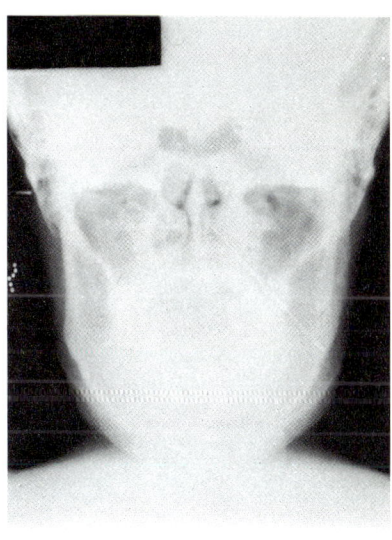
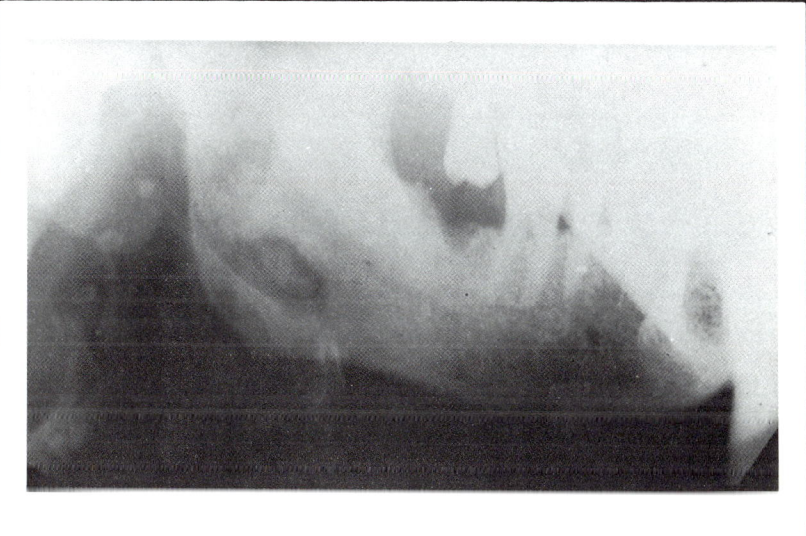

53

Fig. 59. A facial sinus due to chronic periapical suppuration. The sinus mouth is drawn in by fibrous contracture to the mandible and pus discharges intermittently. *(522.7X)*

Fig. 60. An intra-oral view reveals the offending tooth roots. Such sinuses may persist for years, to dry up only when the causative tooth is removed. The sinus must also be excised in order to separate the skin from the mandible, and the wound is then closed in layers.

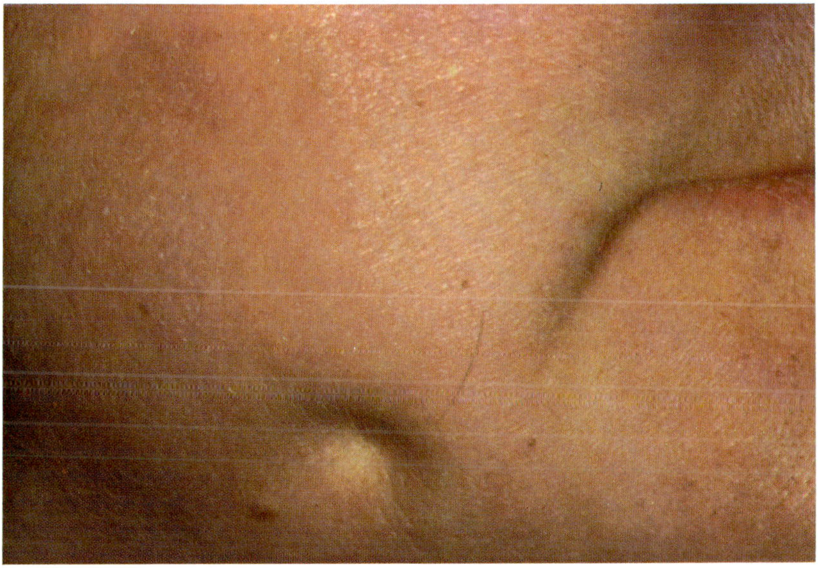

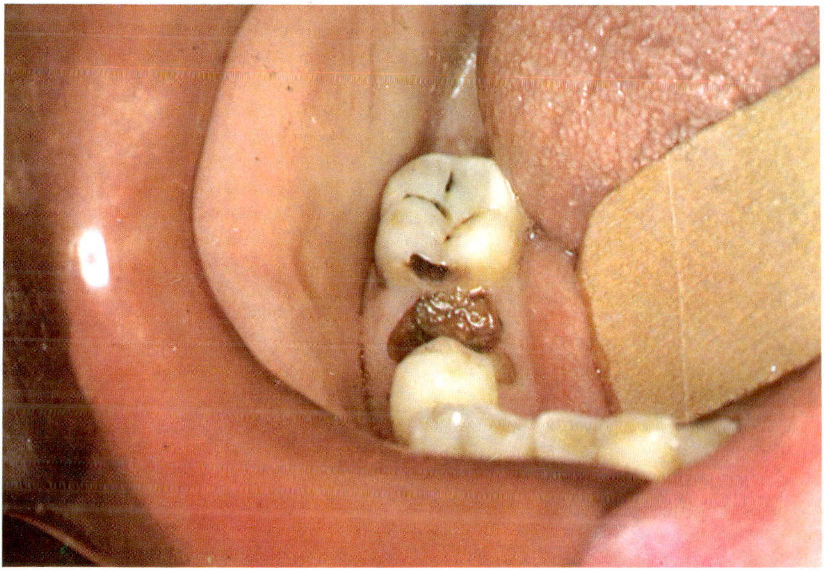

55

Fig. 61. The x-ray of the roots in the preceding case shows periapical radiolucency due to chronic infection. *(522.6X)*

Fig. 62. Chronic periapical abscess on an upper right deciduous central incisor. Note the rampant caries in the whole deciduous dentition. *(522.6X)*

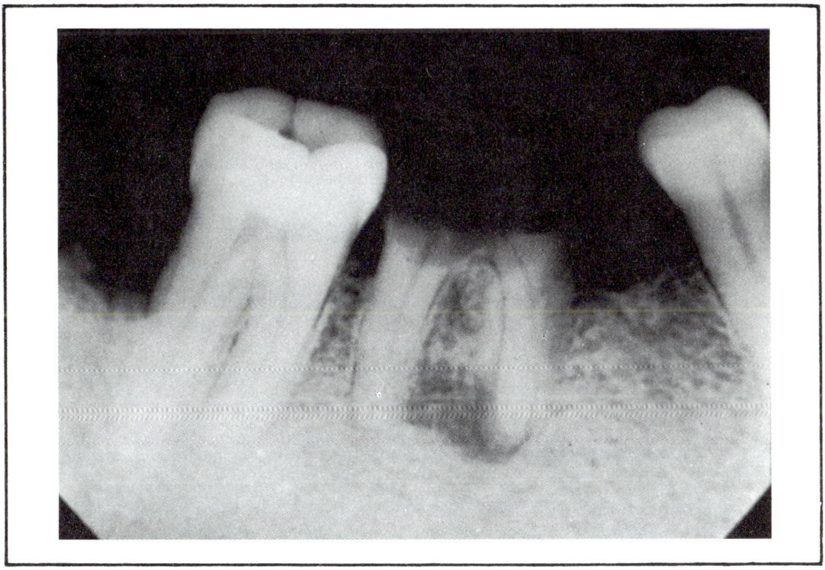

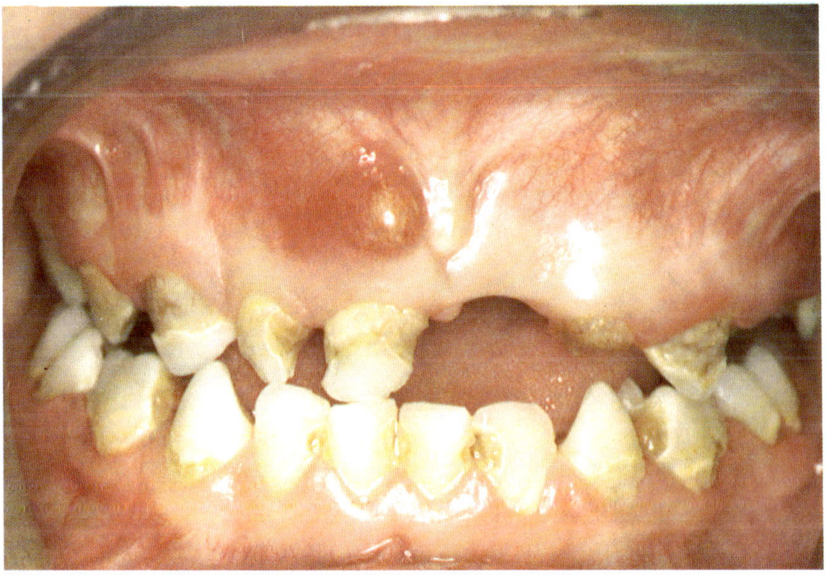

57

Fig. 63. A sinus draining a chronic focus of periapical infection associated with a dead upper left lateral incisor. This tooth is the commonest source of dental abscesses in the anterior part of the maxilla and pus from it commonly points palatally. In this particular case, the canine was also non-vital. *(522.7X)*

Fig. 64. Suppuration in the parotid gland is associated with pre-auricular swelling, pain and pus emerging from the parotid duct as here. *(527.2X)*

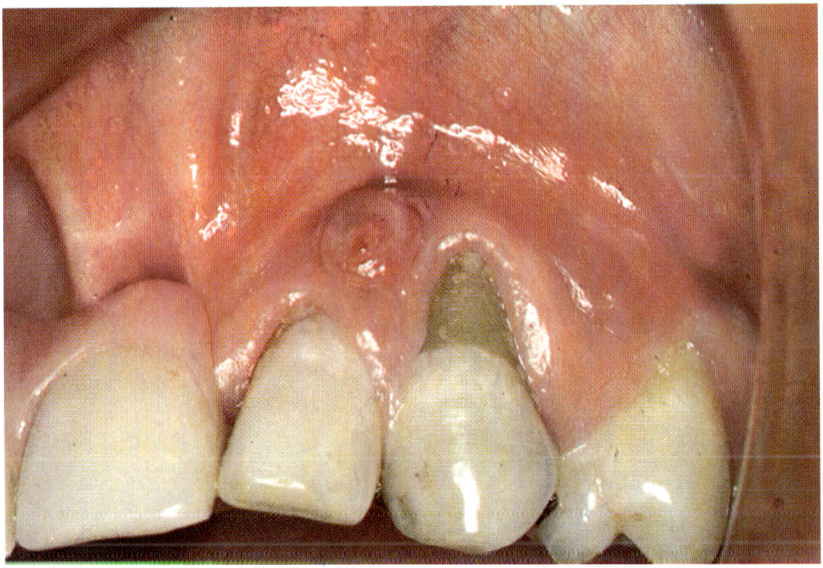

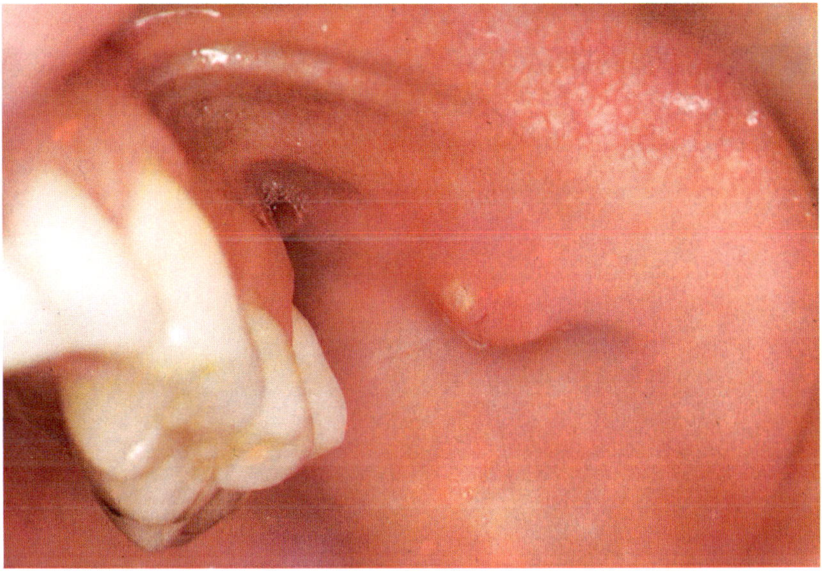

59

Fig. 65. Patient with acute parotitis. Note the outward displacement of the left ear. The swelling is tender but the overlying skin is not inflamed. *(527.2X)*

Fig. 66. This youth has a branchial cyst which must be distinguished from upper deep cervical lymphadenopathy. The swelling is painless and persistent, although it may fluctuate in size. *(745.4X)*

Fig. 67. A median mental sinus. This is always due to periapical suppuration on the lower incisor teeth. *(522.7X)*

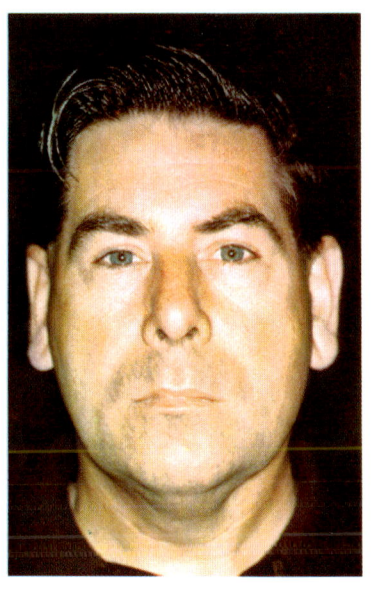
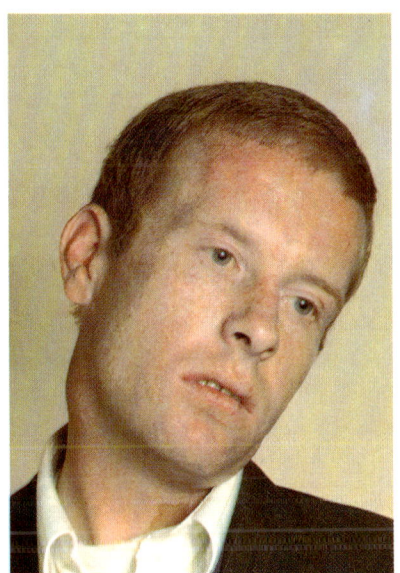

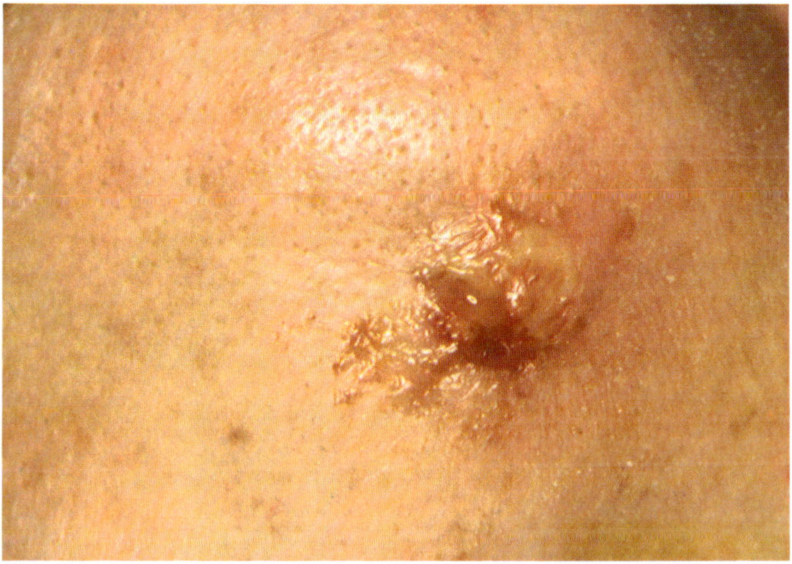

Fig. 68. Here are multiple sinuses on the alveolus following tooth extraction. These are typical of osteomyelitis. The oral mucosa is inflamed. The history is one of persistent pain and swelling, and mental anaesthesia is an early feature. *(526.41)*

Fig. 69. The x-ray shows widespread bone destruction; this is a case of subperiosteal osteomyelitis. *(526.41)*

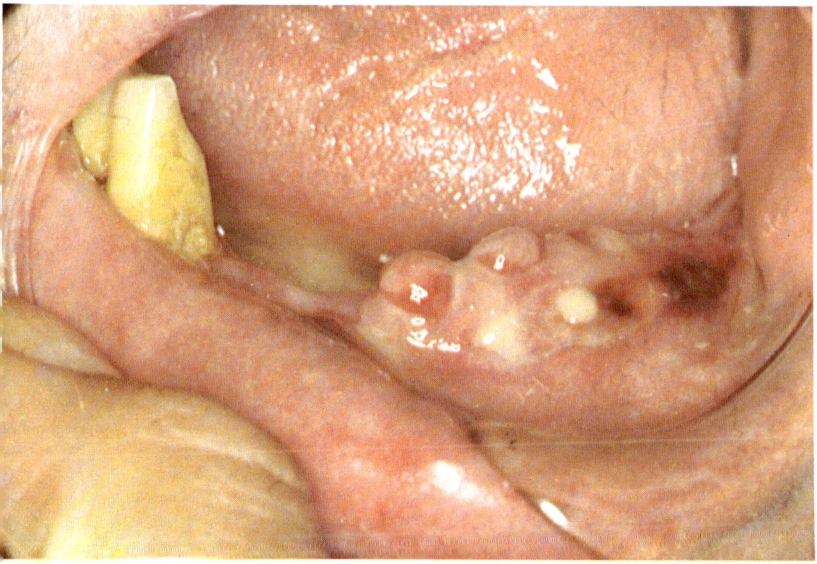

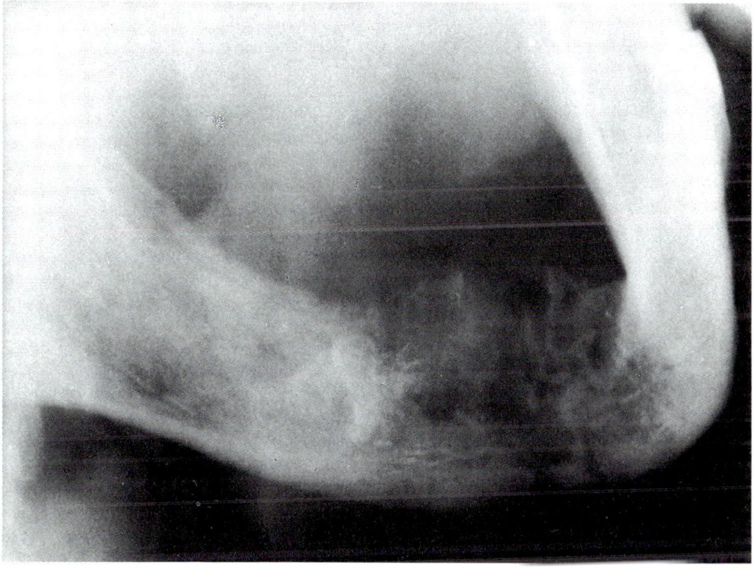

63

SECTION THREE: **THE TEETH**

Fig. 70. This x-ray shows the typical features of intra-medullary osteomyelitis. There is a large sequestrum involving the lower border. There were intra-oral and extra-oral sinuses in this case. *(526.41)*

Fig. 71. This wisdom tooth shows a sharply marked yellow line due to the administration of tetracycline at the age of 15 years or so; a not uncommon finding in patients who have received the drug after puberty for acne vulgaris. All antibiotics in the tetracycline group cause staining of the developing teeth, and the discoloration is permanent. Therefore, to avoid an aesthetic problem, these drugs should not be prescribed for pregnant women during the second and third trimester, or for children below the age of eight years. *(520.93)*

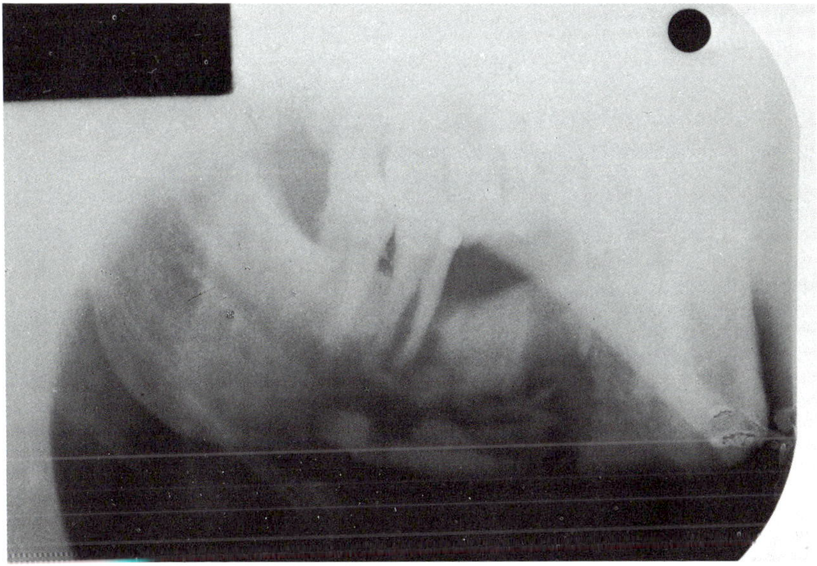

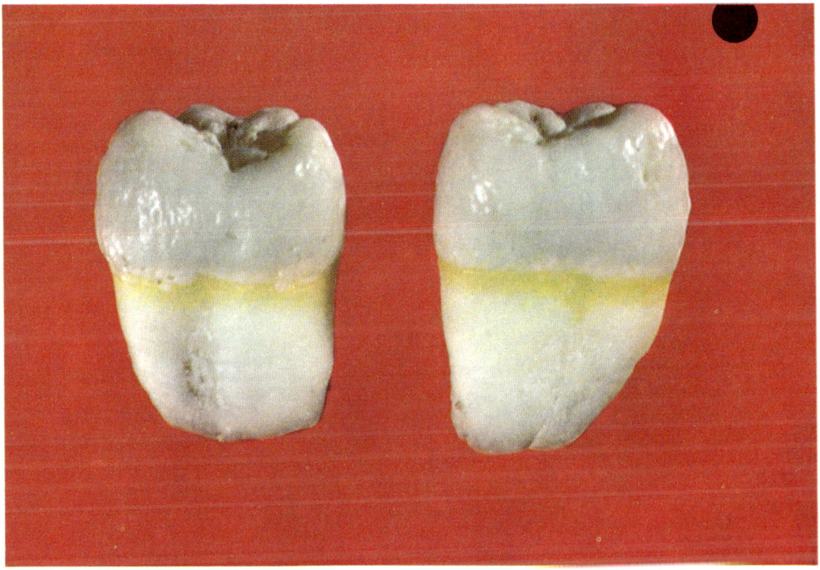

65

Fig. 72. Hutchinson's incisors. Note the barrel shape and the incisal notching due to the deletion of the central tubercle of the teeth; part of the ravages of congenital syphilis. *(090.51)*

Fig. 73. Teeth malformed and resembling those of congenital syphilis. This, however, is a case of simple hypoplasia. Note that the central tubercles are present. *(520.29)*

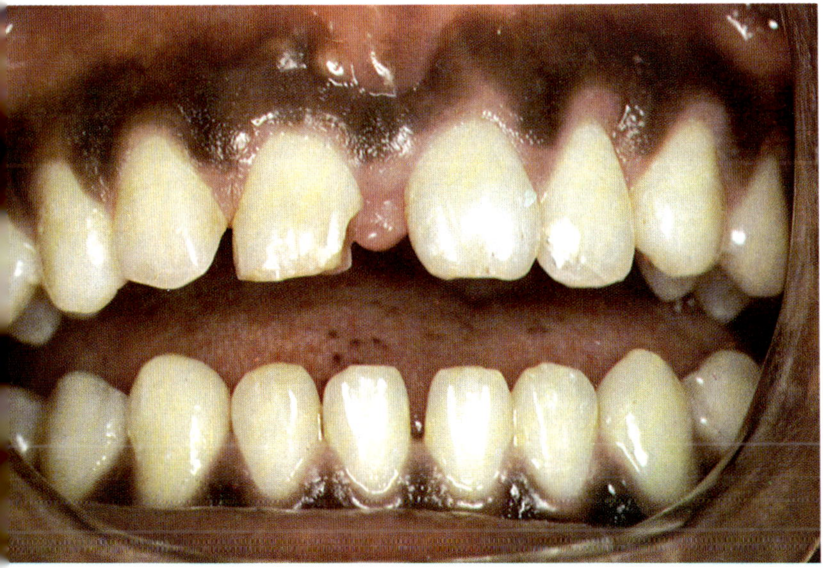

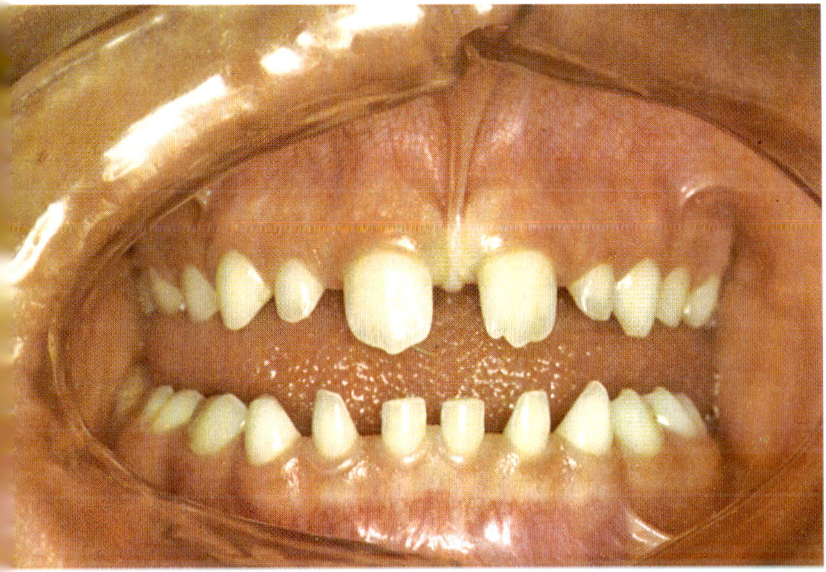

67

Fig. 74. These teeth are typical of fluorosis where the level of fluoride in the drinking water is high (3–5 p.p.m.). They are heavily stained by absorption of constituents of the diet into hypoplastic enamel. Notwithstanding which, such teeth exhibit remarkable caries resistance due to their chemical composition. *(520.30)*

Fig. 75. These teeth are severely stained due to the habit of chewing betel; the staining may be due in part to tobacco which is often chewed with the betel. The habit of chewing tobacco (with betel) causes oral keratosis with, subsequently, a very high incidence of squamous-cell carcinoma. *(521.72)*

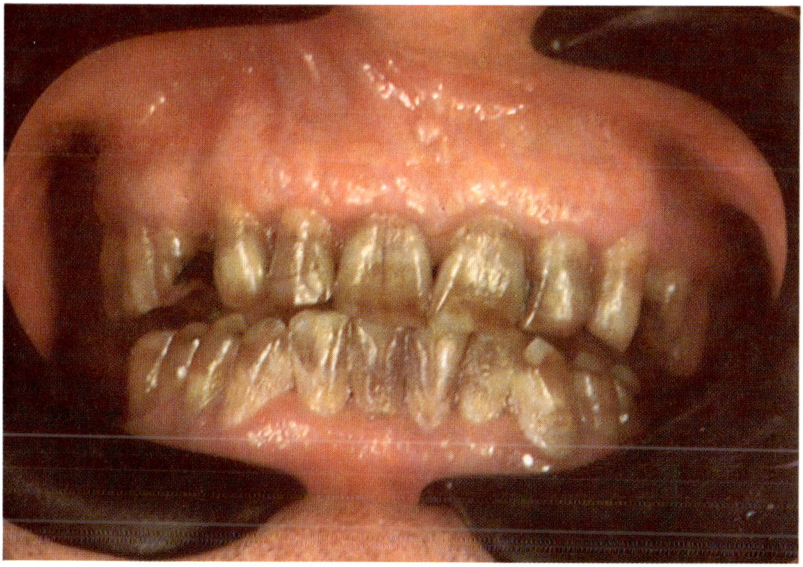

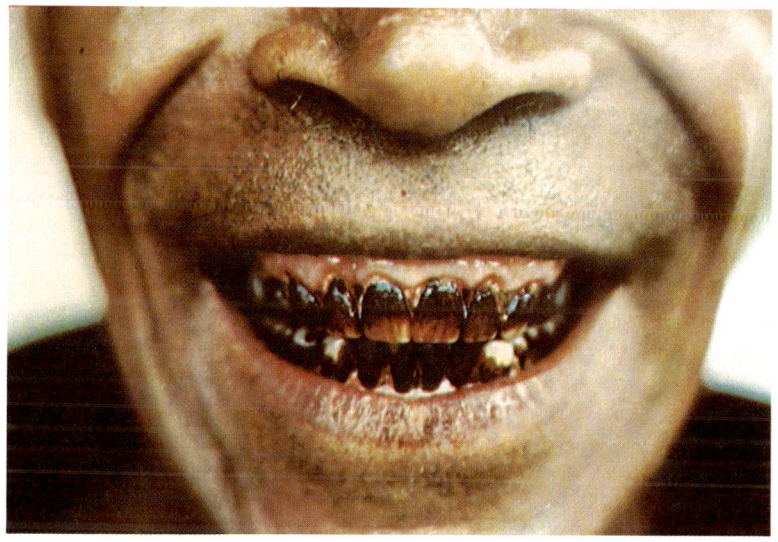

Fig. 76. Abrasion of a tooth due to repeated opening of hair-grips. *(521.21)*

Fig. 77. Severe toothbrush abrasion of the teeth. Note that the patient brushes only the left side of his mouth and several teeth have been severed at gum level. To avoid gross misuse of a toothbrush proper instruction in technique should always be dispensed. *(521.20)*

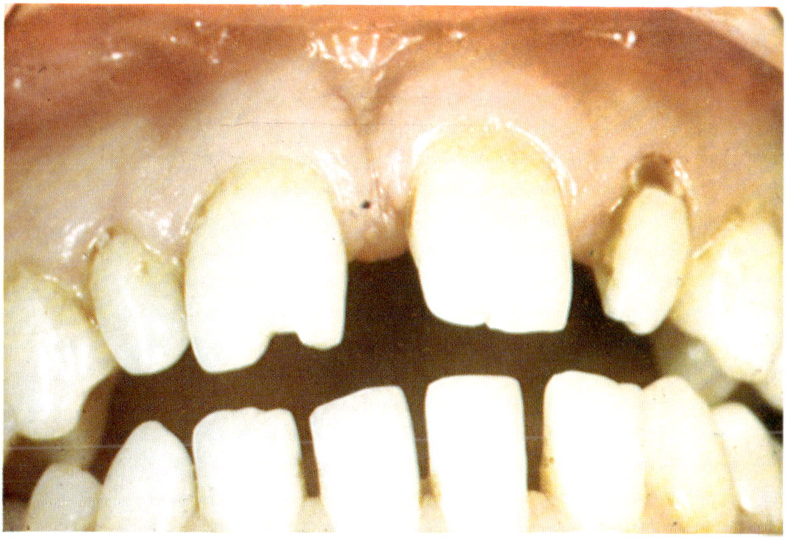

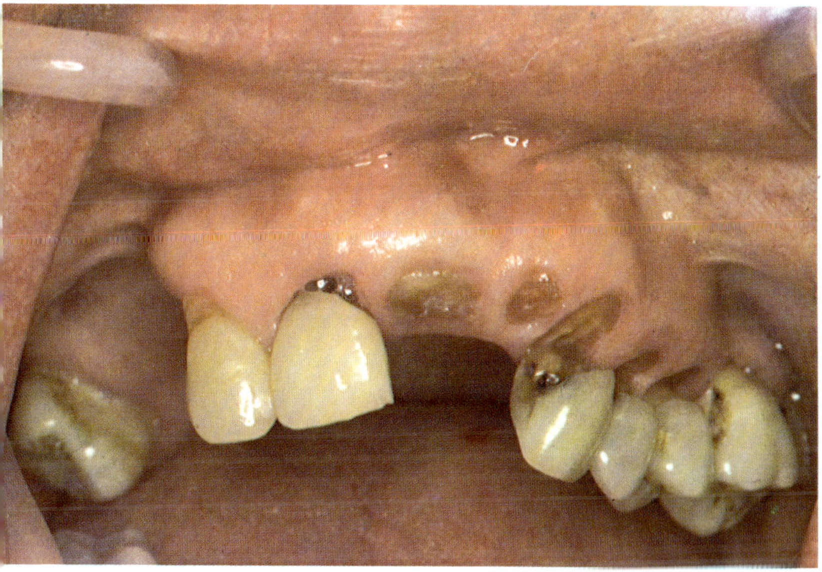

71

Fig. 78. Severe pitted hypoplasia of the upper central incisors of "chronological" type due to severe systemic disturbance at about one year of age. *(520.40)*

Fig. 79. Severe generalised enamel hypocalcification, an inherited defect; but note that the deciduous teeth are not affected. This is a variety of amelogenesis imperfecta. *(520.50)*

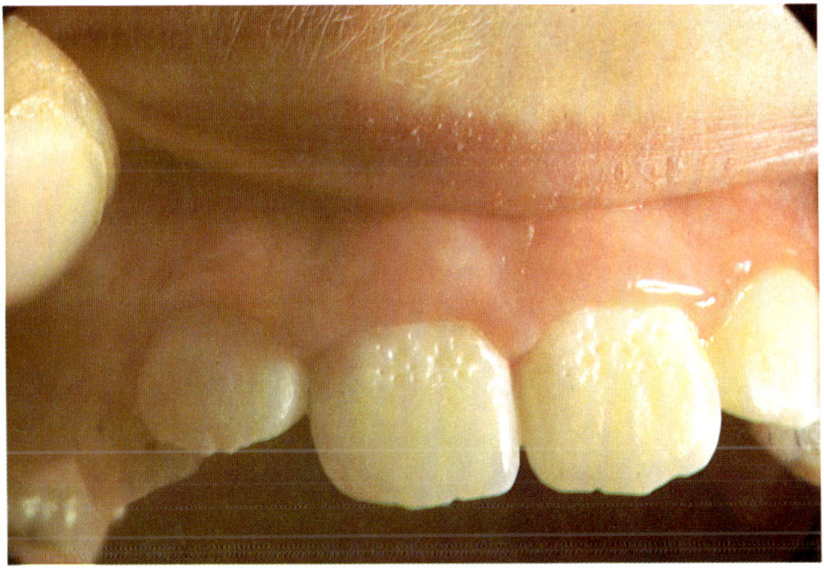

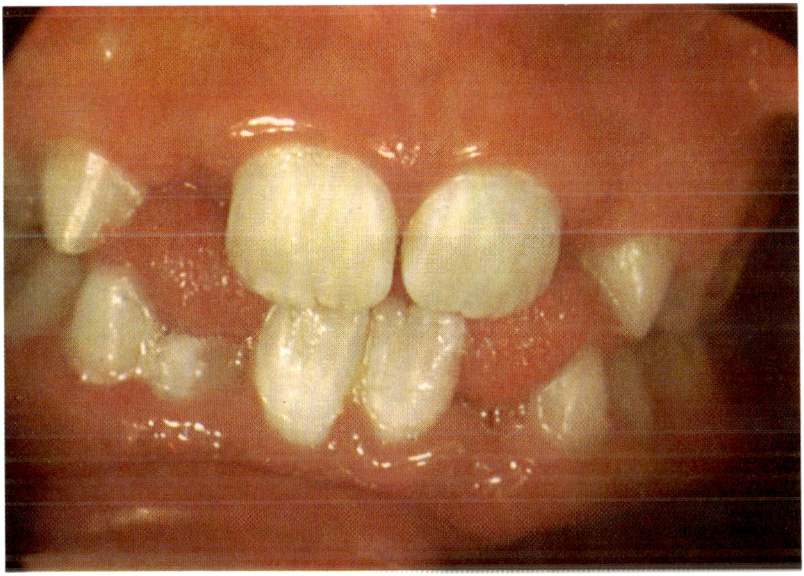

Fig. 80. The same as the previous illustration (**fig. 79**) but here the teeth are more severely involved. *(520.50)*

Fig. 81. "Snow-capped teeth," another form of hypocalcification of the enamel of the incisal third of the teeth, again thought to be a hereditary variant of amelogenesis imperfecta. *(520.50)*

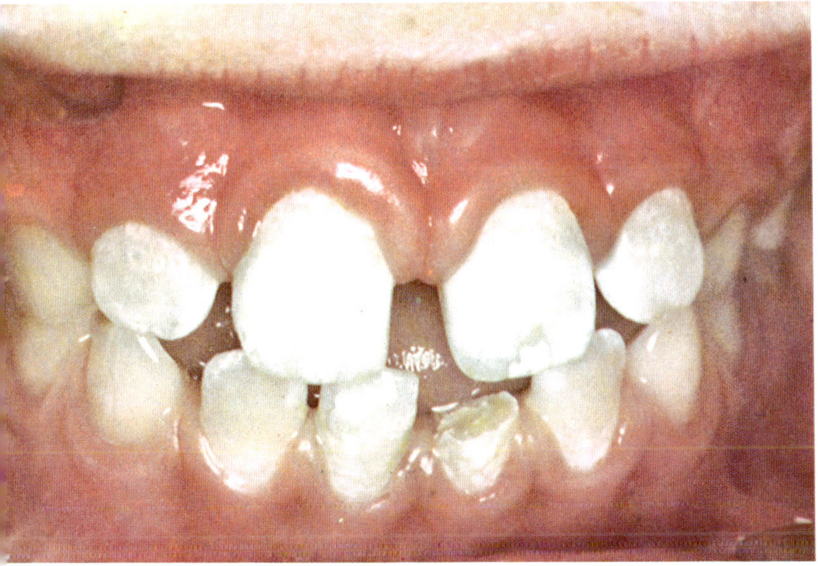

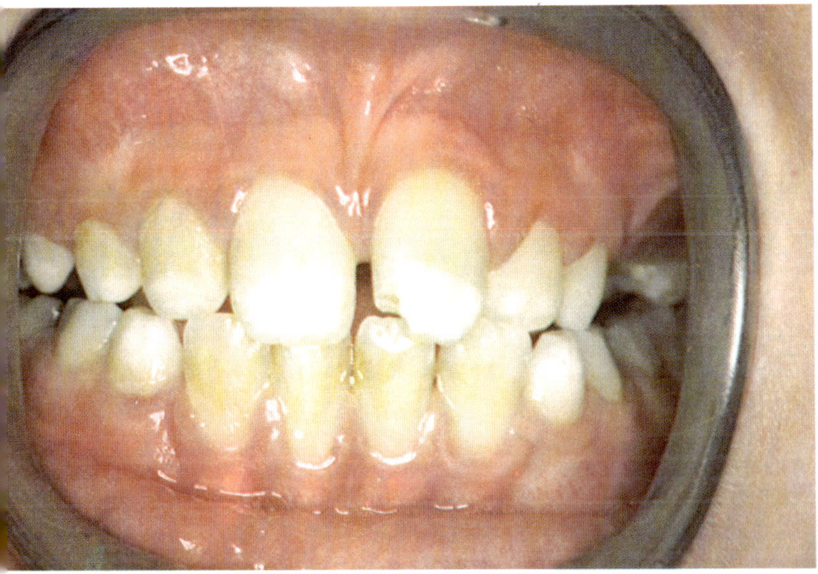

75

Fig. 82. Hereditary dentinogenesis imperfecta which may be associated with osteogenesis imperfecta. The deciduous teeth are also affected. The teeth have a bluish hue on eruption, but the colour rapidly darkens to a deep blue-grey or brown. Enamel subsequently flakes off the teeth, which leads to extensive occlusal wear since the dentine is softer than normal, while the pulp chambers are progressively obliterated by vasodentine. *(520.51)*

Fig. 83. Staining of teeth which have been rendered non-vital by trauma; the discoloration is due to blood pigments aspirated into the dentinal tubules. *(N873.75)*

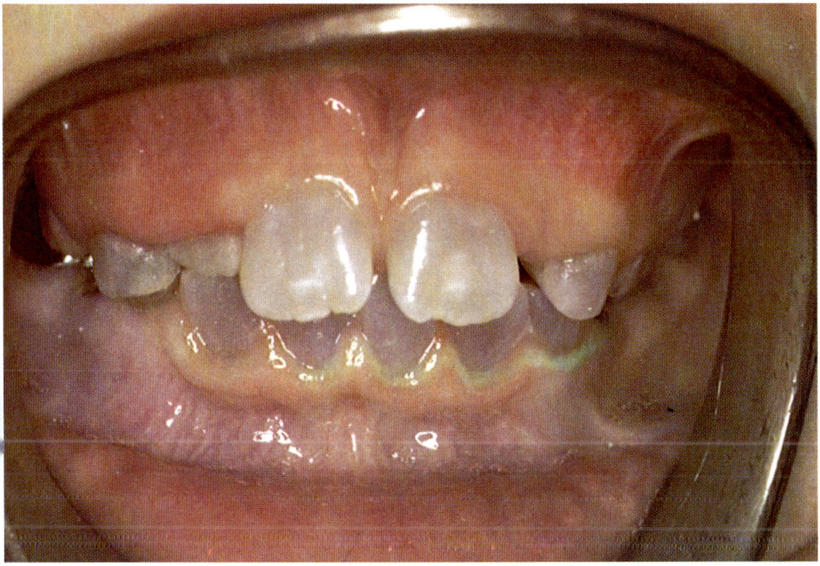

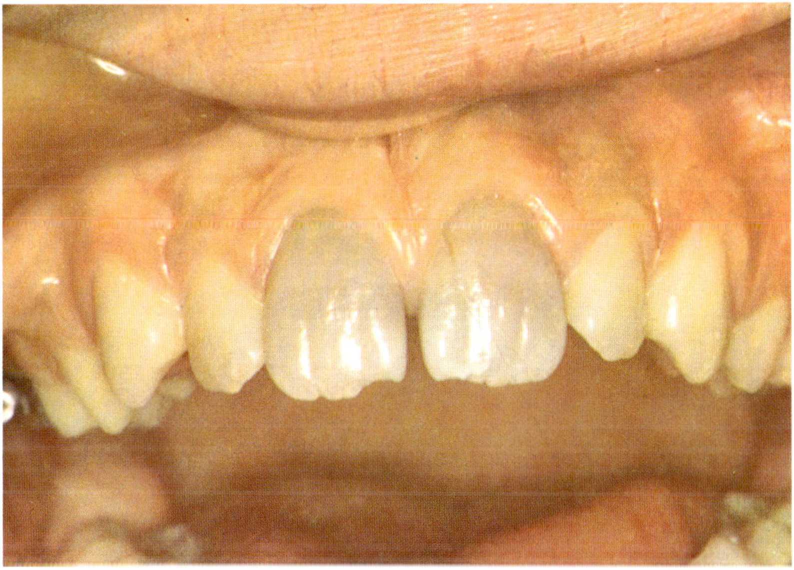

Fig. 84. Dentinogenesis imperfecta, again of the deciduous dentition. *(520.51)*

Fig. 85. Tetracycline staining of the teeth due to the drug having been given to the patient's mother during pregnancy. The drug is permanently absorbed into calcifying dental tissues. *(520.93)*

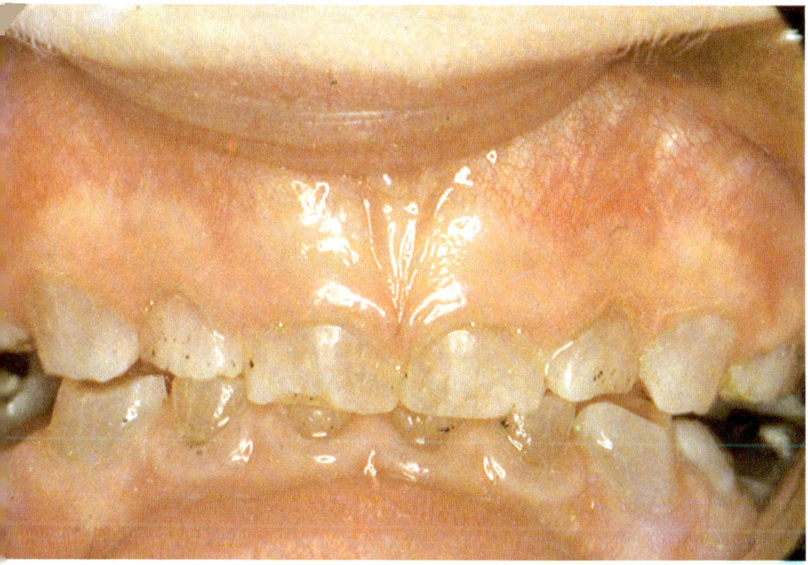

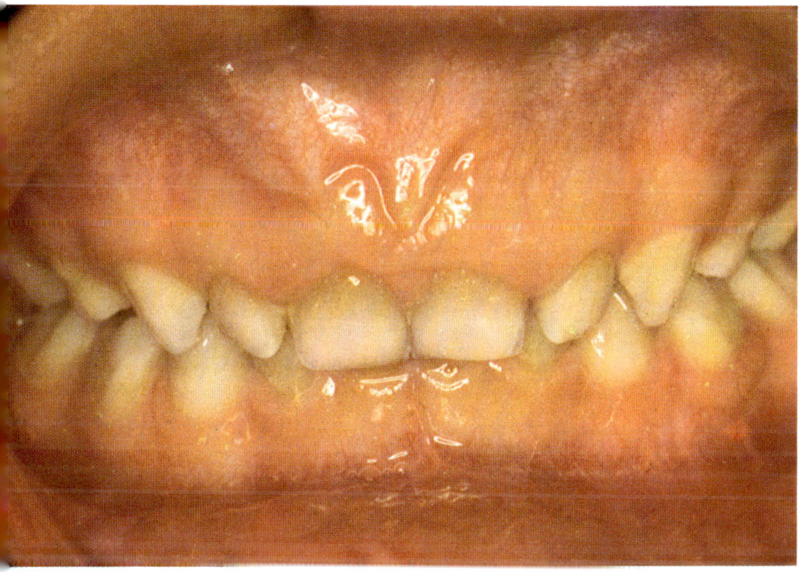

79

Fig. 86. Severe enamel hypoplasia of hereditary type. The enamel has largely worn off the incisors and the remainder is stained by extrinsic absorption (amelogenesis imperfecta). *(520.50)*

Fig. 87. Severe enamel (and dentine) hypoplasia due to rickets. This is frequently associated with an anterior open bite. *(265.10)*

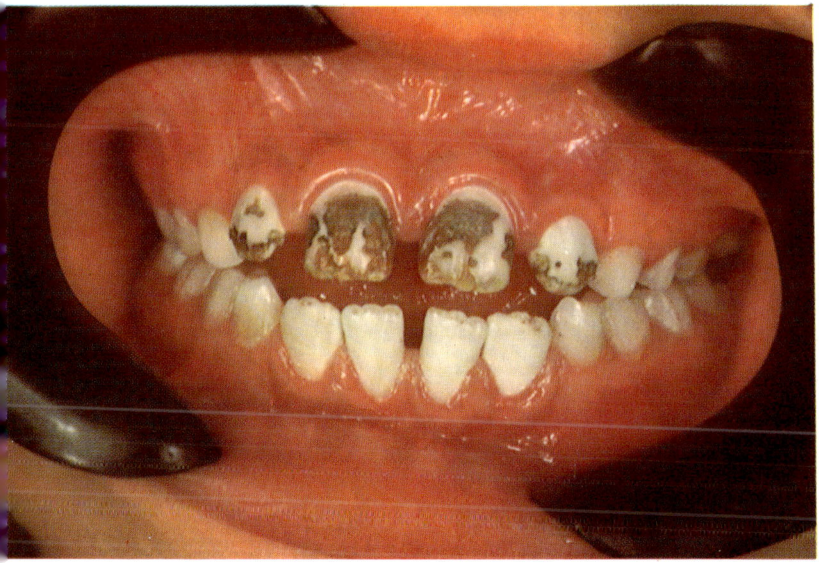

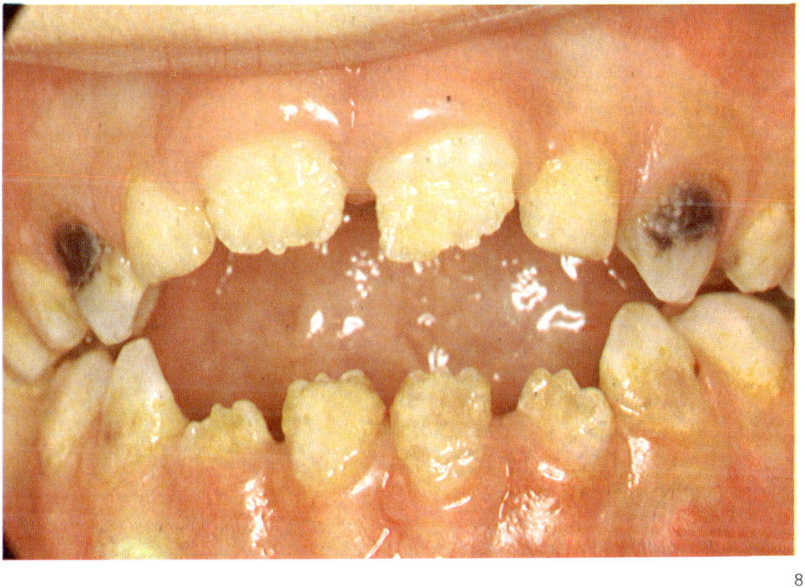

81

Fig. 88. Connation of the upper right central incisor. This abnormality is probably due to fusion of its germ with that of a supernumerary tooth. *(520.23)*

Fig. 89. Connation of the upper central incisors. The condition, apart from being unsightly, may cause overcrowding of adjacent teeth. *(520.23)*

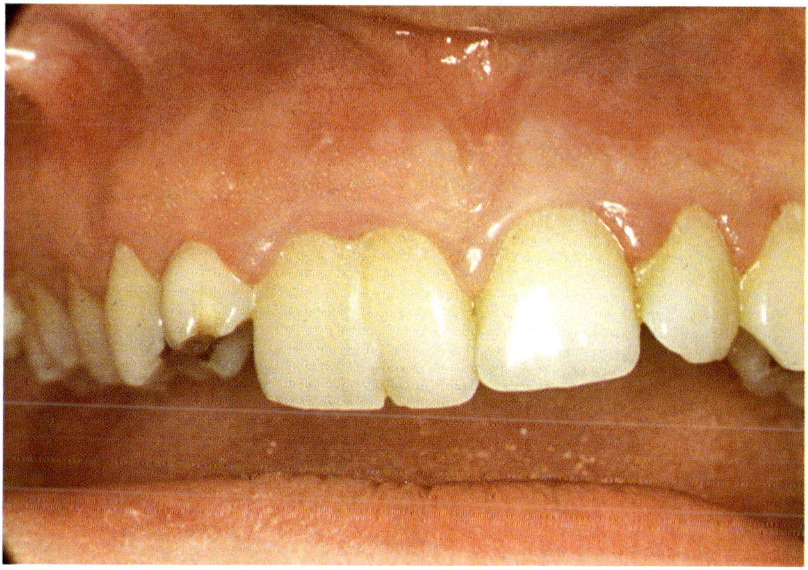

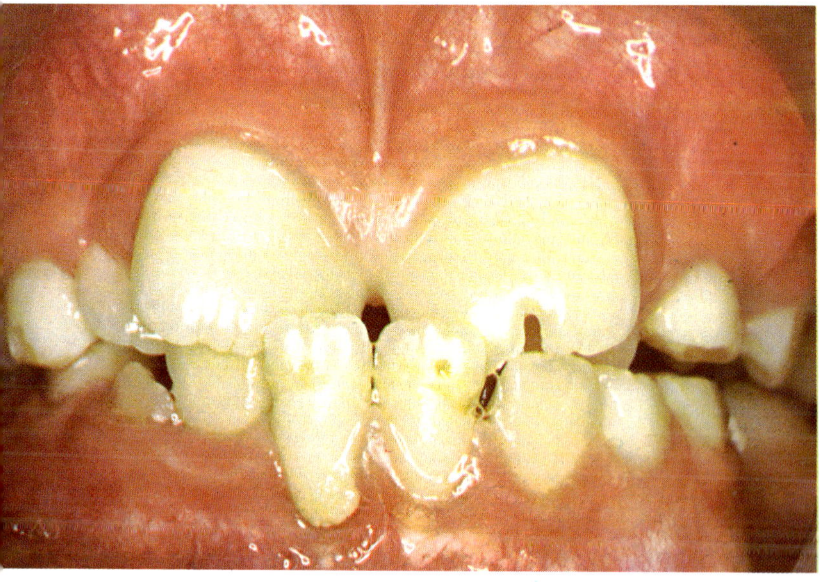

83

Fig. 90. A supernumerary tooth erupting in the palate. The upper incisor region is the most frequent site of accessory teeth. They are usually conical but fail to erupt, and they also impede the eruption of the central incisors or cause a median diastema. *(520.10)*

Fig. 91. Simple overcrowding due to a disproportion between tooth size and the space available for the correct alignment of the teeth. *(524.30)*

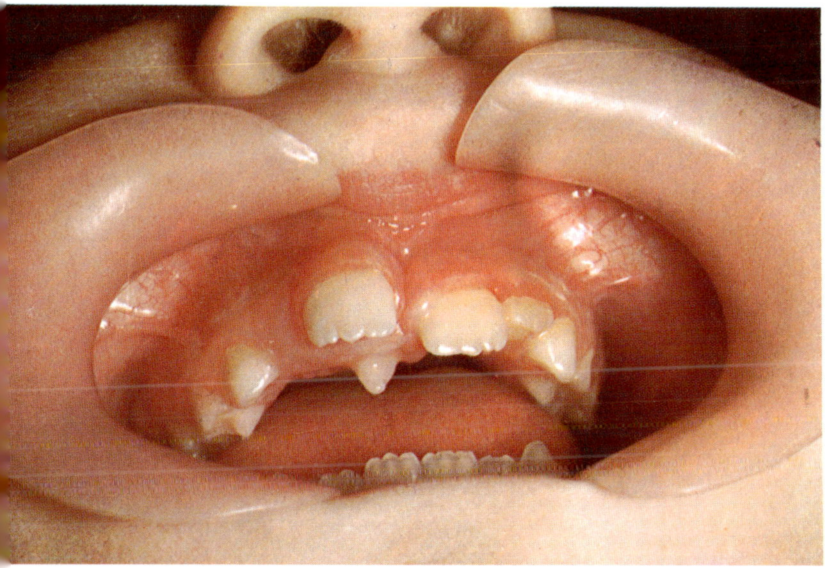

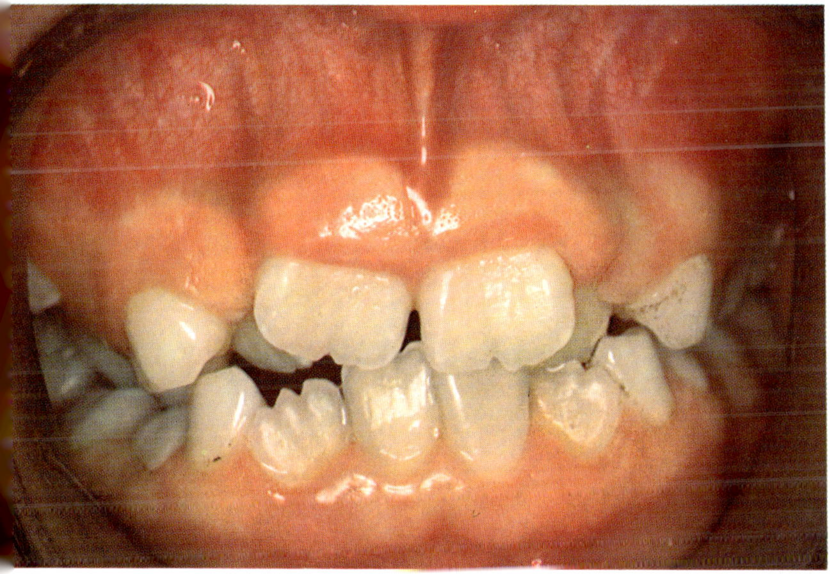

85

Fig. 92. Undue retention of upper deciduous incisors with the succedaneous teeth erupting labially; this is a rather unusual event. *(520.63)*

Fig. 93. Here the upper left first deciduous molar is retained and its mesial root exposed, as a result of chronic periapical infection. The upper left first premolar is erupting. Note that the upper left central incisor is absent. *(520.63)*

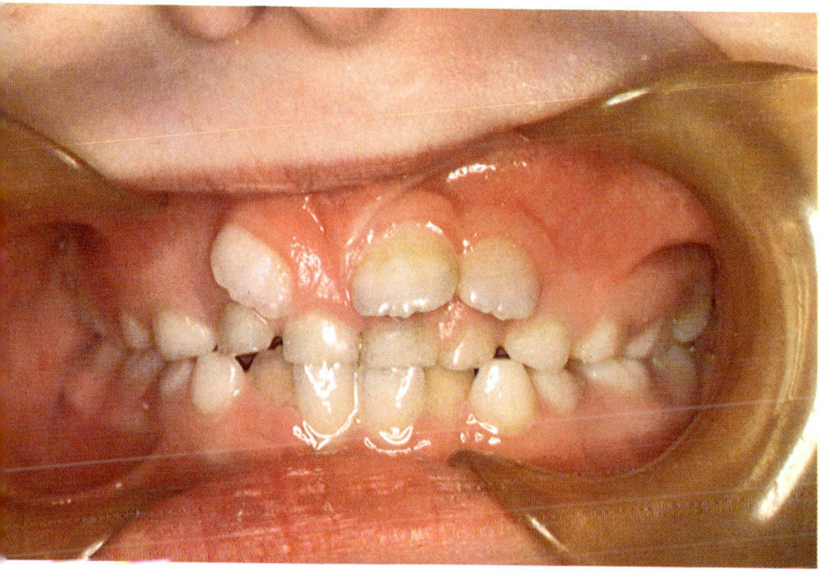

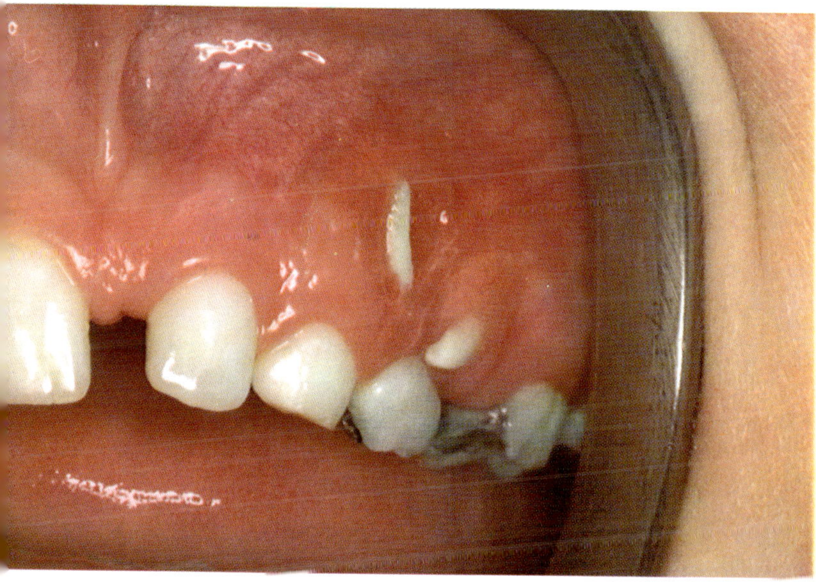

07

Fig. 94. "Pink spot" of the upper left lateral incisor due to idiopathic internal resorption of the tooth so that the pulp chamber occupies a much greater size than usual. *(521.41)*

Fig. 95. A pulp polyp of the left mandibular second molar. This is, in essence, a pyogenic granuloma derived from pulp tissue exposed by acute caries. The granuloma receives an epithelial cover from desquamated oral mucosal cells. *(522.05)*

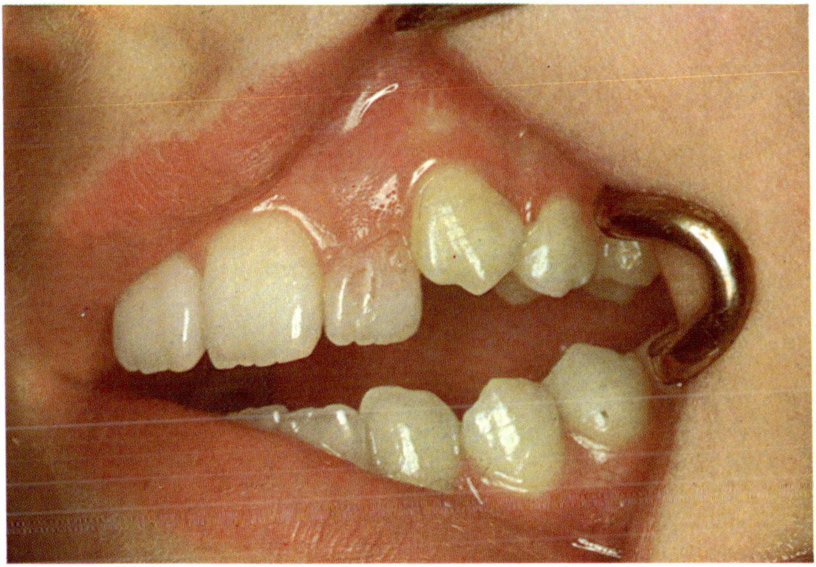

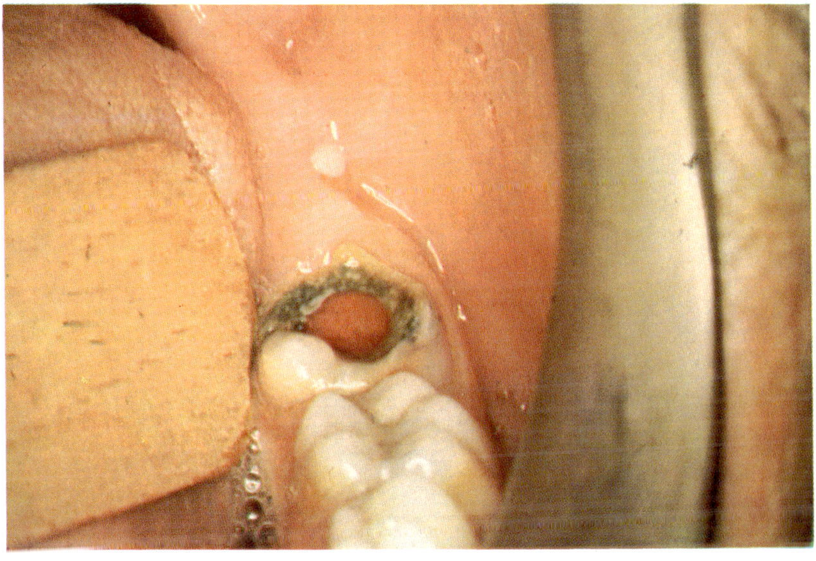

Fig. 96. Fractured incisors. This is a very common pattern of injury in children with prominent upper incisors (Cl.2. division 1 malocclusion). Here the fracture involves enamel and dentine only and the pulps are vital. *(N.873.71)*

Fig. 97. More extensive fracture of the crown with pulpal exposure and necrosis and subsequent discoloration of the dentine. *(N873.72)*

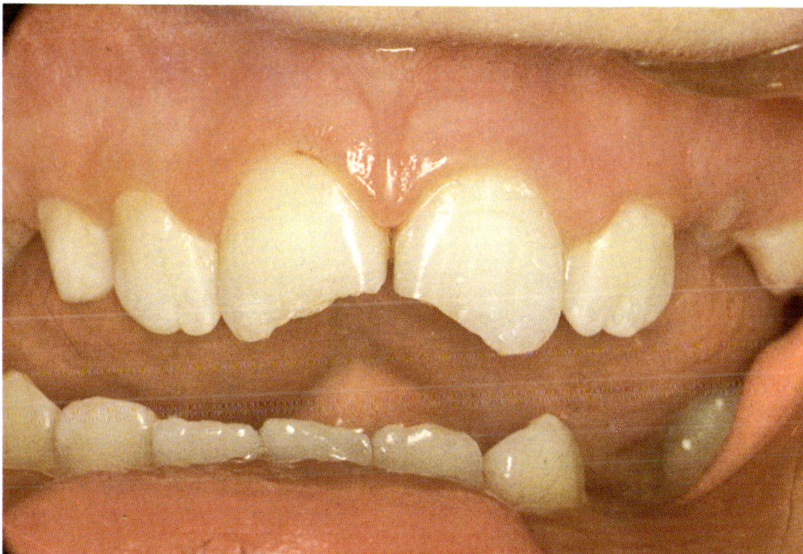

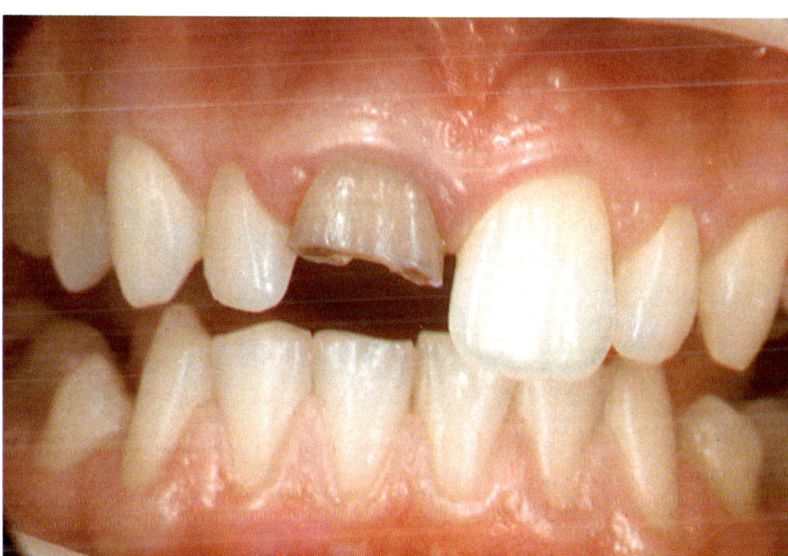

91

Fig. 98. A similar fracture of the crown as in the last case, but immediately after the injury to demonstrate exposure of the pulp. The loss of tooth substance is always greater on the palatal than on the labial surface. *(N873.72)*

Fig. 99. Complete avulsion of the upper left central incisor. If the patient cannot produce the tooth, x-rays of the chest and open soft tissue wounds are required to ensure that it is not in these sites. *(N873.78)*

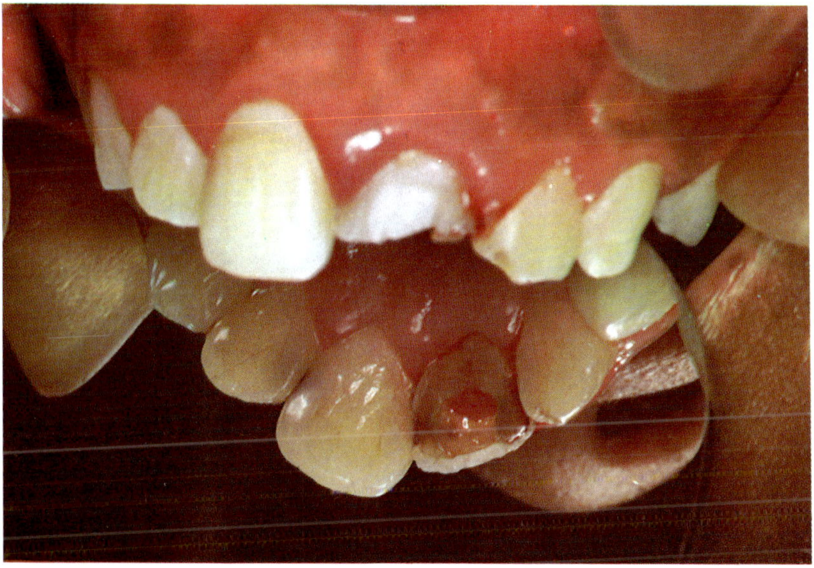

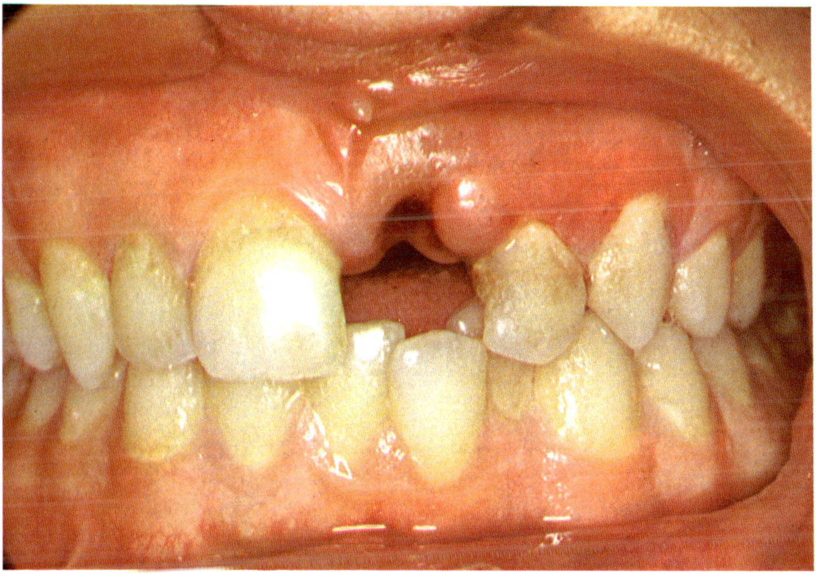

93

Fig. 100. A submerged lower first deciduous molar with retention of the upper left second deciduous molar and an erupting upper left first premolar. *(521.6X)*

Fig. 101. An x-ray of a submerged mandibular second deciduous molar. In this case, as is frequent, the succeeding tooth is absent. A submerged tooth is a deciduous molar which has undergone some resorption of its roots but then becomes ankylosed to bone. Growth in height of the adjacent alveolus and the eruption of neighbouring teeth produces the illusion of progressive depression of the affected tooth below the normal occlusal level. *(521.6X)*

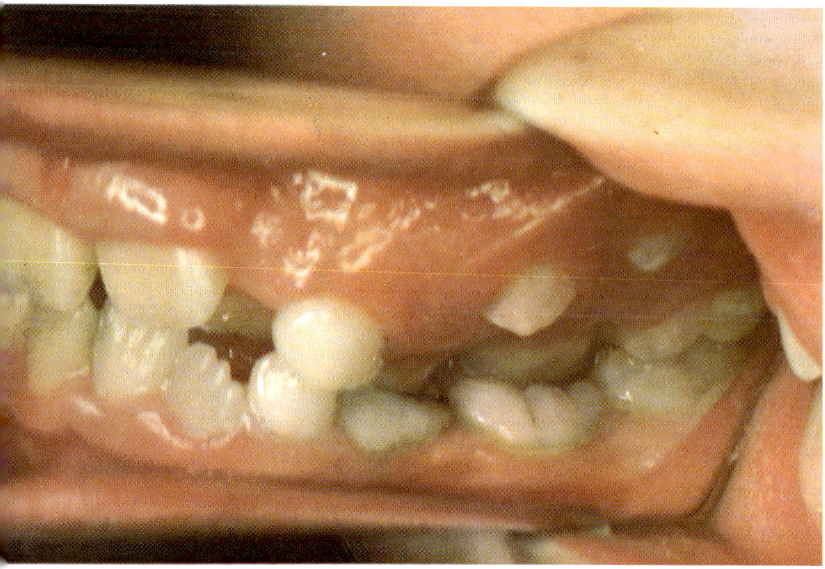

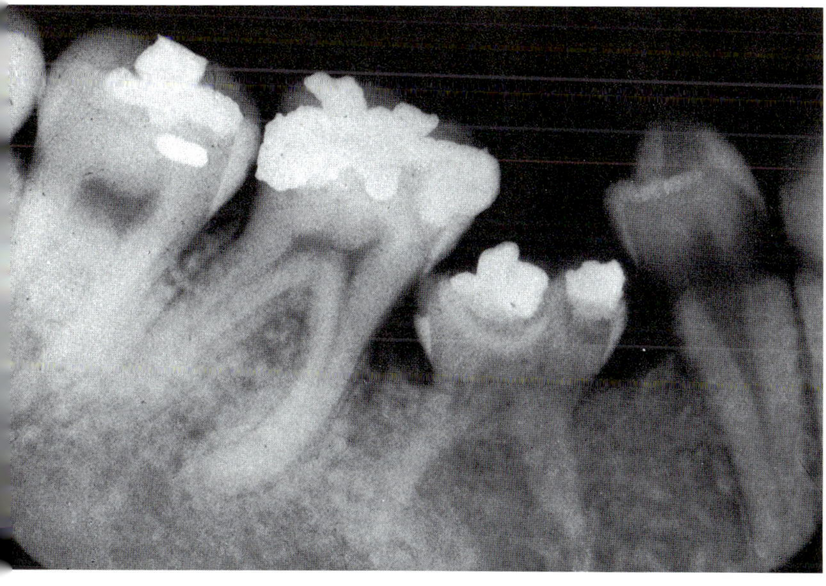

95

Fig. 102. A severe dento-alveolar malocclusion due to thumb-sucking; observe that the distortion of the alveolus is asymmetrical. Note also the poor oral hygiene and extensive green stain on the gingival third of the tooth crowns. *(524.22)*

Fig. 103. Extensive black staining of the deciduous teeth. This type of discoloration is difficult to remove and is associated with a resistance to dental caries. Like green stain, its cause is unknown. *(523.60)*

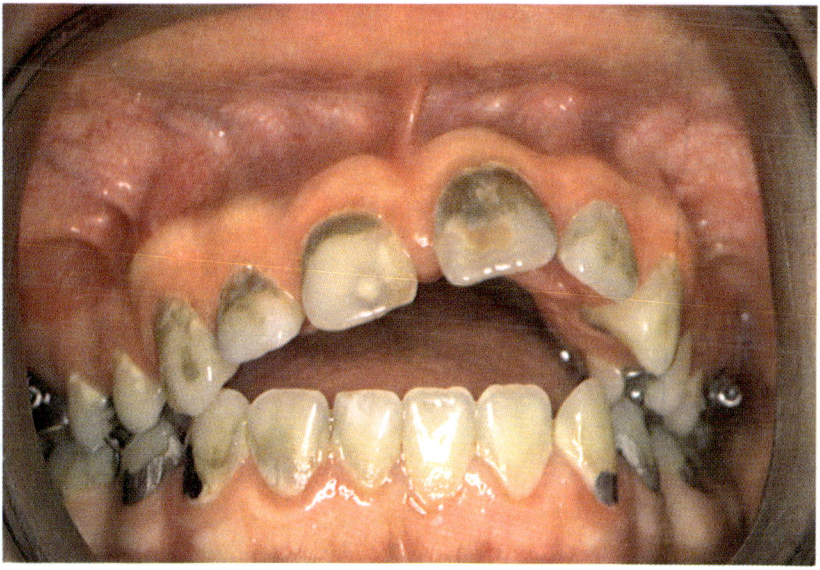

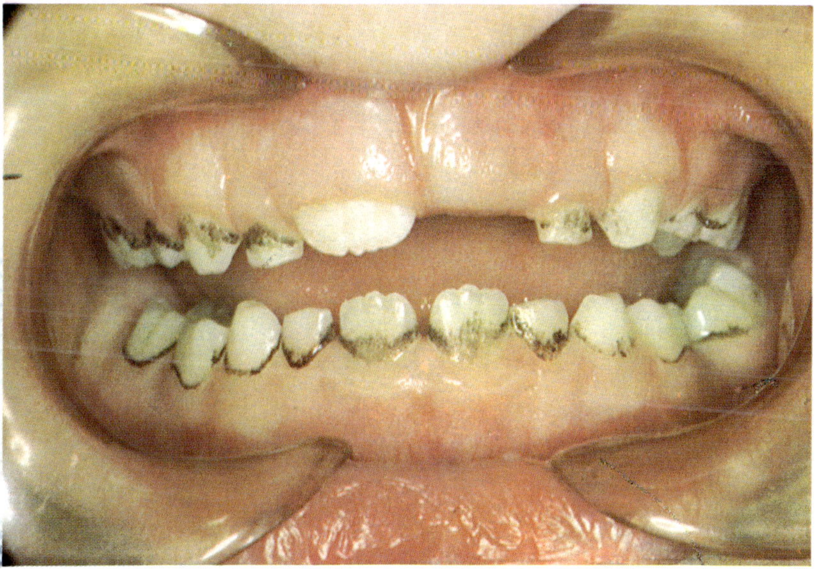

97

Fig. 104. Rampant caries in a child. Note the decay of the lower incisors which are most resistant to attack. Caries is a scourge of "civilisation". *(521.00)*

Fig. 105. This picture shows a normal upper right second molar and a very large corresponding tooth with extensive hypercementosis. Hyperplasia of the cementum covering the root is one of the causes of difficulty in the extraction of teeth. *(521.5X)*

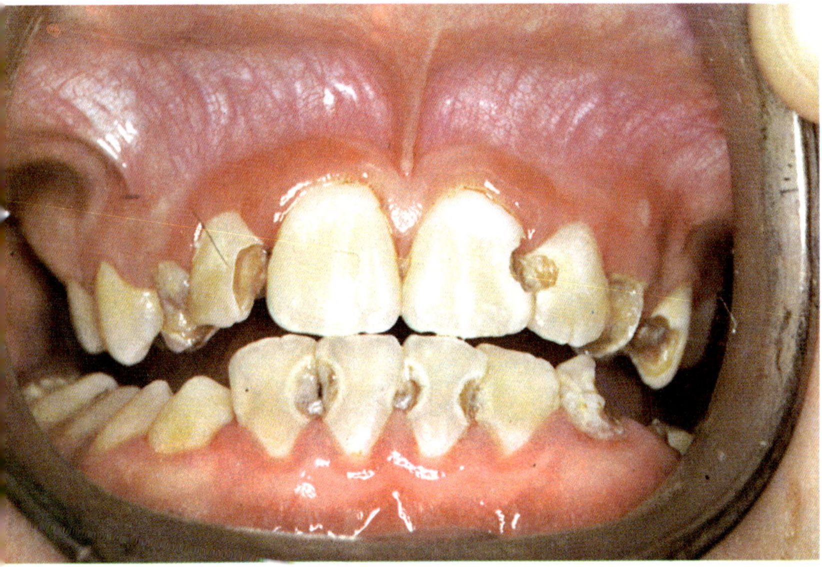

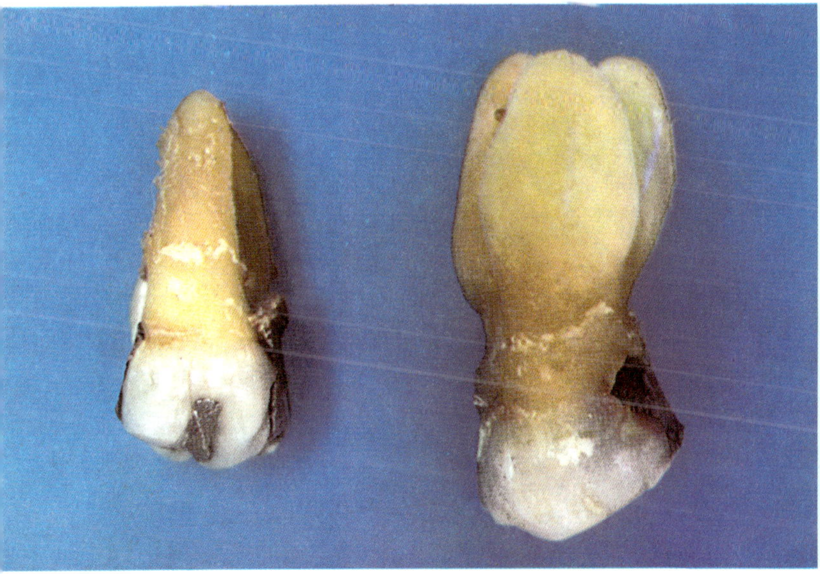

99

Fig. 106. This x-ray shows a recent extraction socket (of the upper right first molar) complicated by dislodgement of the distobuccal root into the antral cavity. This accident occurs frequently and an operation should be arranged at the earliest opportunity to retrieve the displaced root and effect surgical repair of the oro-antral fistula. Early operation will prevent the occurrence of irreversible chronic changes in the mucosa of the maxillary sinus. *(N998.60)*

Fig. 107. Another x-ray film of displaced roots, this time of the left mandibular third molar. They have slipped into the lax soft tissue space medial to the mandible — the so-called sublingual pouch. Immediate surgical retrieval of these fragments is important before they move into the lateral pharyngeal space and cause severe infection. *(N998.99)*

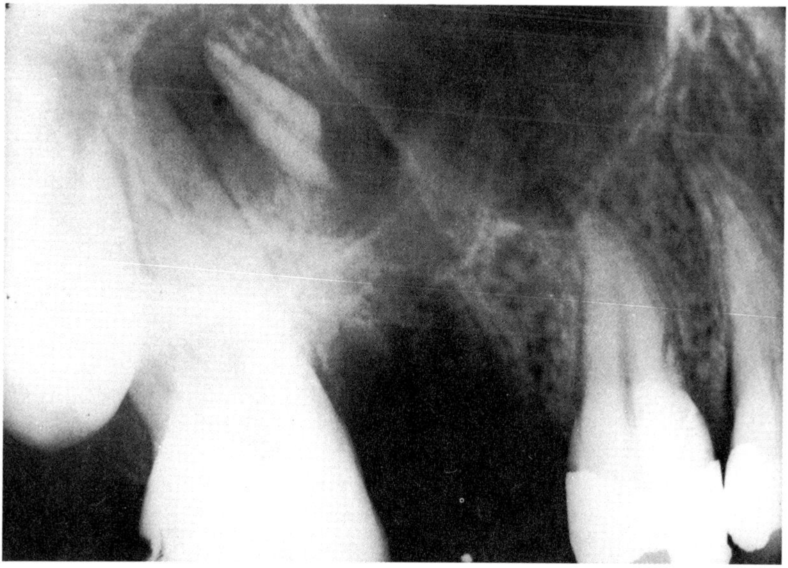

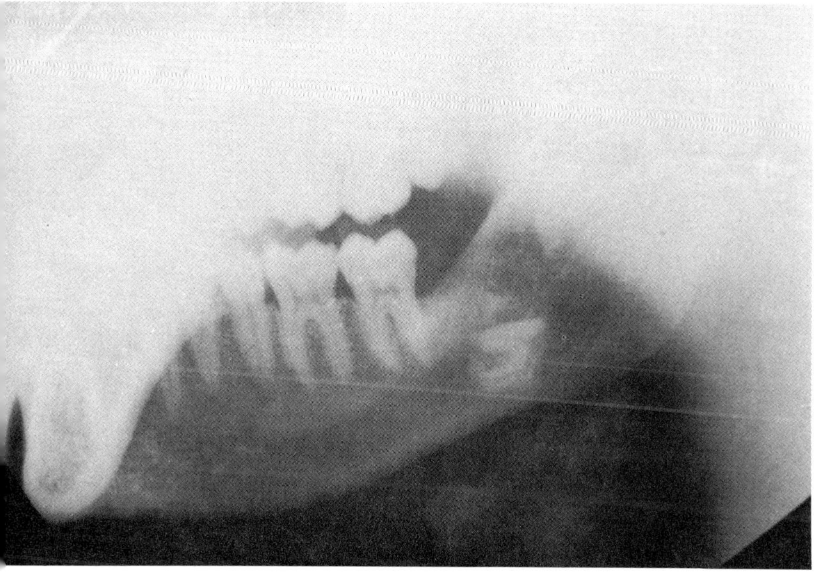

101

SECTION FOUR: **THE GINGIVAE**

Fig. 108. This is the normal gingiva of the lower incisor region. Observe light-pink, stippled attached gingival mucosa with sharply pointed interdental papillae.

Fig. 109. In contrast, this view shows a mass of supragingival calculus which is due to an accumulation of debris, and poor oral hygiene. Destruction of parodontal tissue is extensive and most of these teeth are loose. *(523.64)*

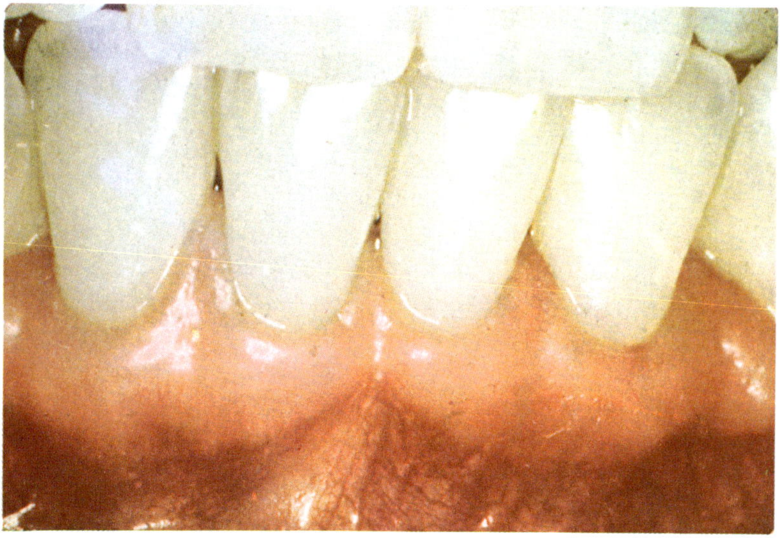

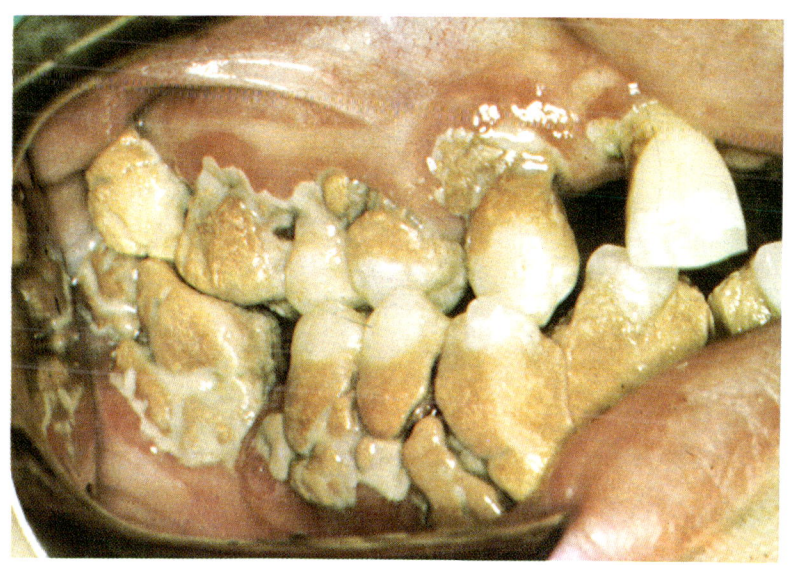

Fig. 110. Marginal gingivitis. Note that the papillae are principally involved and the inflammation has made them smooth and shiny. In the region of the lower left second incisor, the inflammatory process has extended around the whole of the attached gingiva. *(523.10)*

Fig. 111. Rather more severe and extensive marginal gingivitis. *(523.10)*

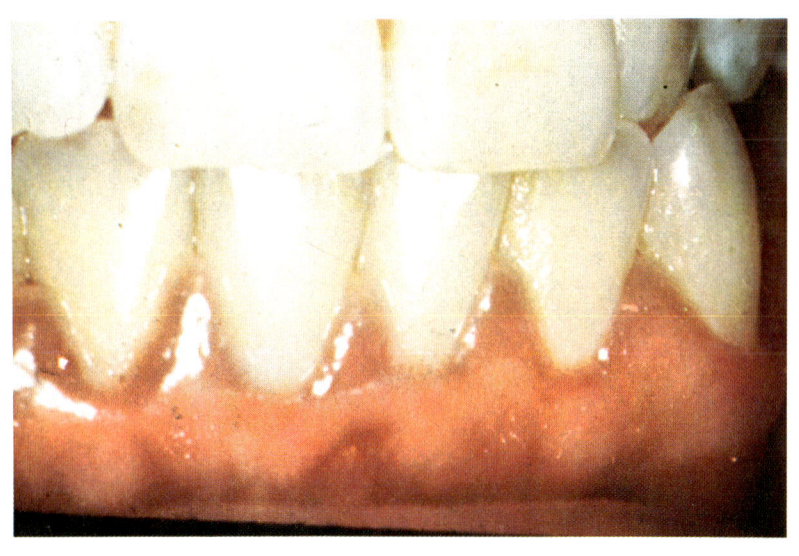

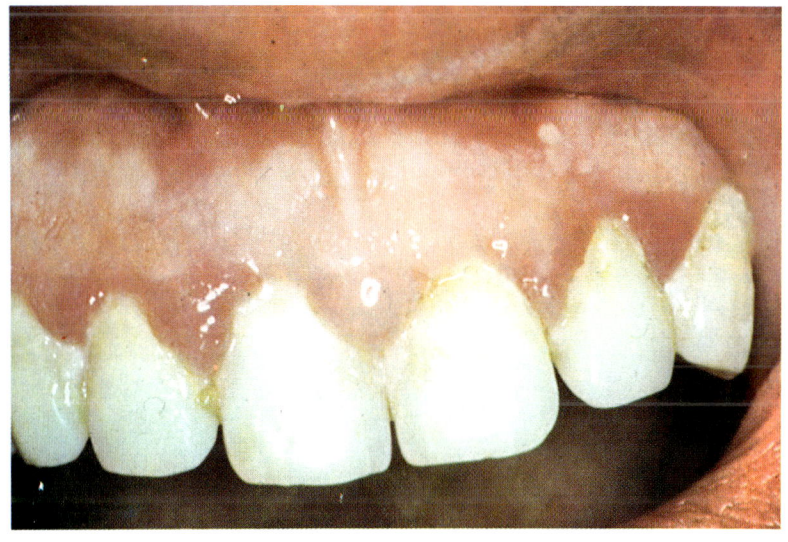

Fig. 112. Mild hyperplastic gingivitis of the upper anterior region which typifies persistent mouth breathing. *(523.11)*

Fig. 113. In this case there is marked severe gingivitis with granulation tissue proliferating around the marginal gingiva. This appearance often occurs in puberty and pregnancy and is occasionally seen in patients taking oral contraceptives. *(523.11)*

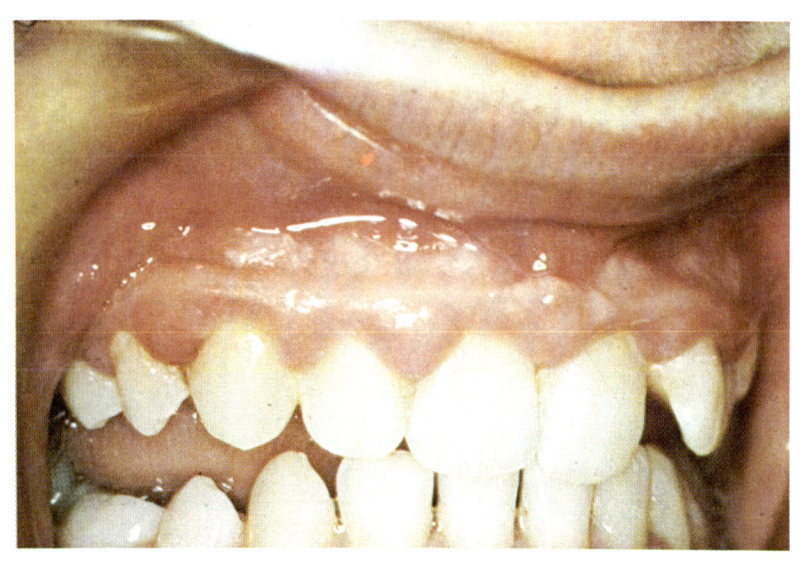

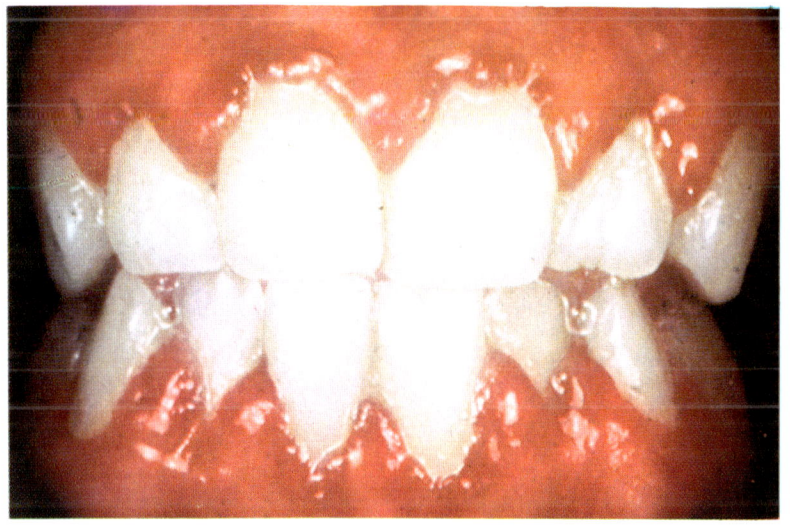

Fig. 114. Chronic periodontal disease showing destruction of interdental papillae and sub- and supra-gingival calculus. *(523.41)*

Fig. 115. Severe gingival recession, which may be an accompaniment of age, even in the absence of inflammation. *(523.21)*

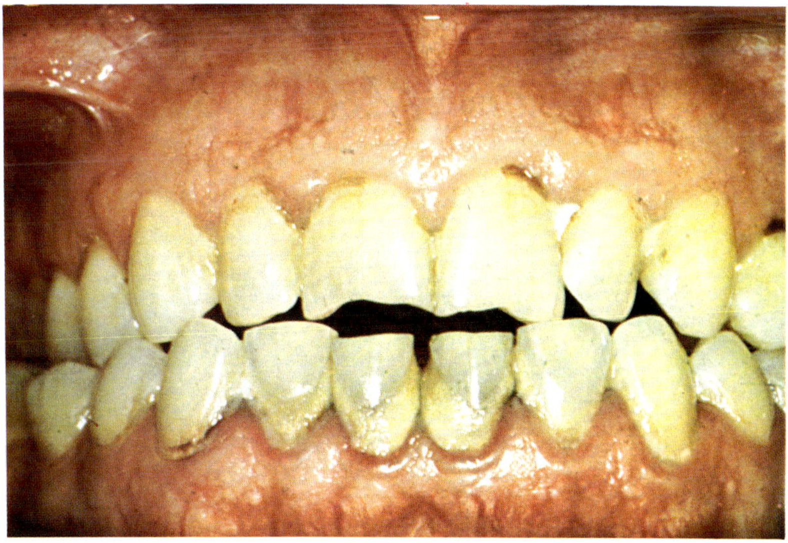

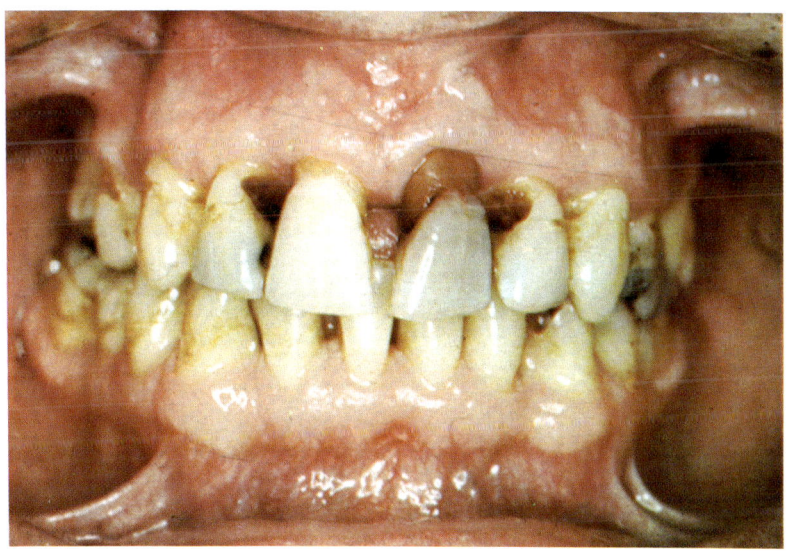

Fig. 116. Acute ulcerative gingivitis — Vincent's gingivitis, probably due to fuso-spirochaetal infection. Note destruction of the interdental papillae, leaving shallow concave ulcers with white necrotic margins and the signs of acute inflammation. A prominent and almost diagnostic feature of the condition is the characteristic halitosis. There may be cervical adenitis. *(101.X0)*

Fig. 117. Acute ulcerative gingivitis of unusual type, being localised to one tooth. Occasionally the lesion spreads over the adjacent attached mucosa in this manner. *(101.X0)*

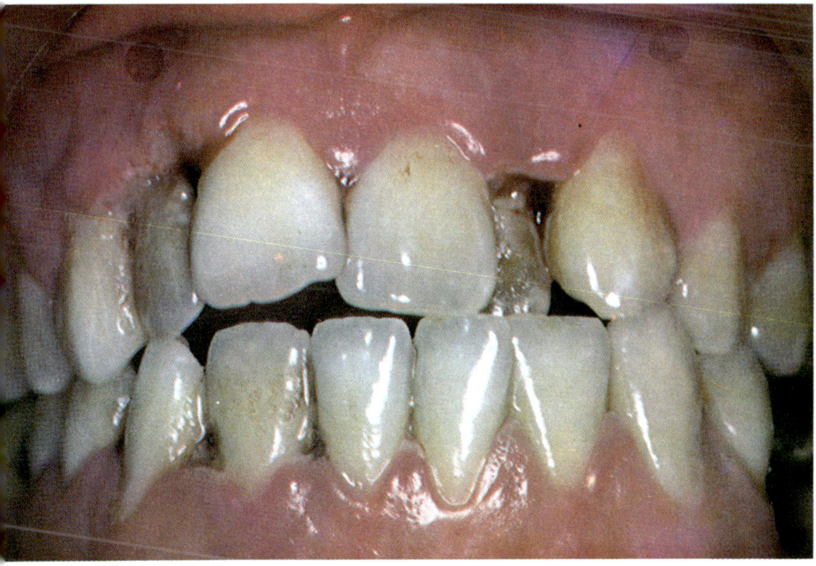

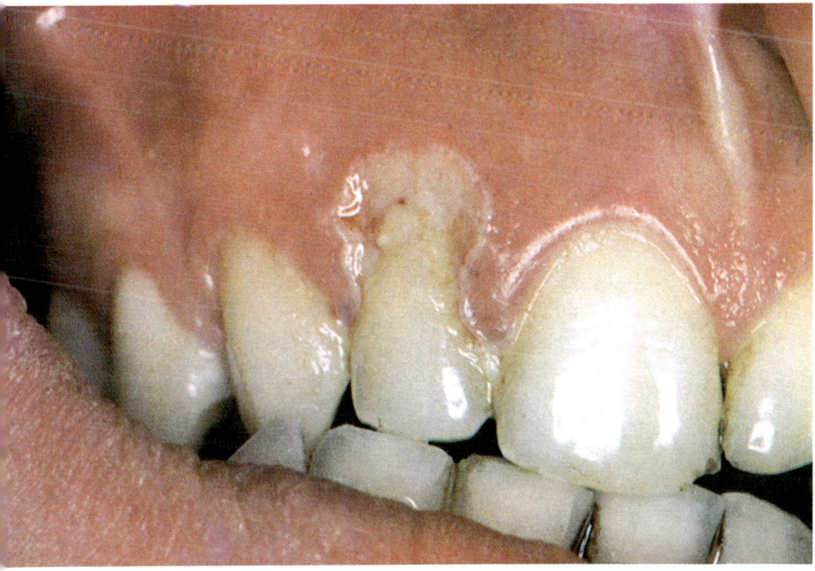

111

Fig. 118. A further example of Vincent's gingivitis with widespread destruction. Note early involvement of the lower incisor region. *(101.X0)*

Fig. 119. In this case the infection has entered a subacute phase with extensive ulceration. *(101.X0)*

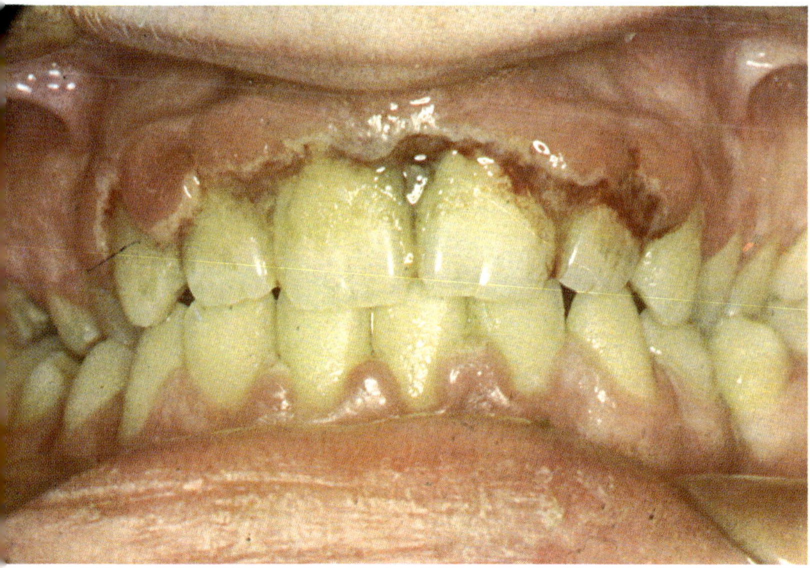

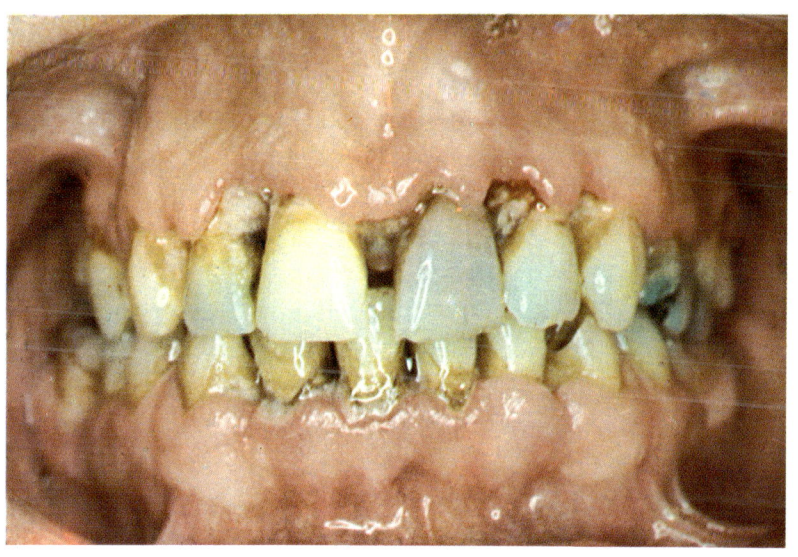

Fig. 120. The typical appearance of the gingivae after acute ulcerative gingivitis. The papillae are absent and the gingival margin is thick and rolled. *(523.20)*

Fig. 121. Chronic hyperplastic gingivitis — in this case due to Epanutin or Dilantin (phenytoin sodium). A similar appearance may result from the exhibition of other drugs (primidone, barbiturates, contraceptive pills), chronic gingivitis or occasionally familial fibromatosis. *(N.966)*

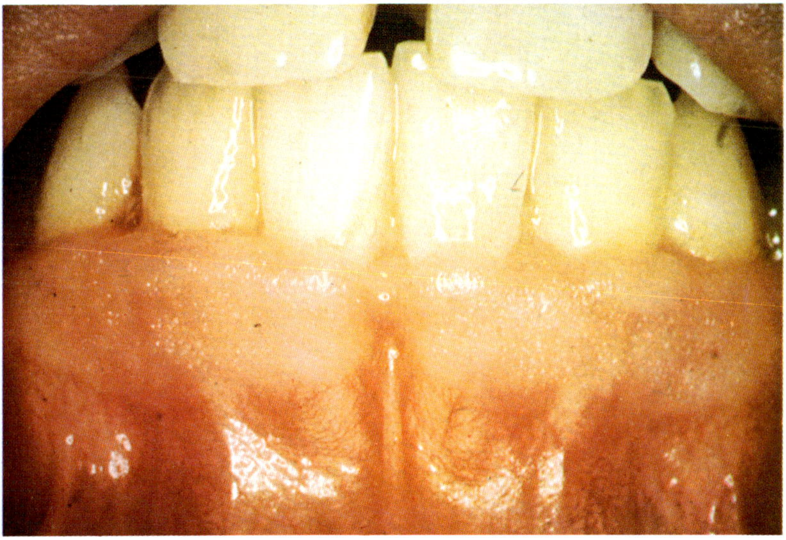

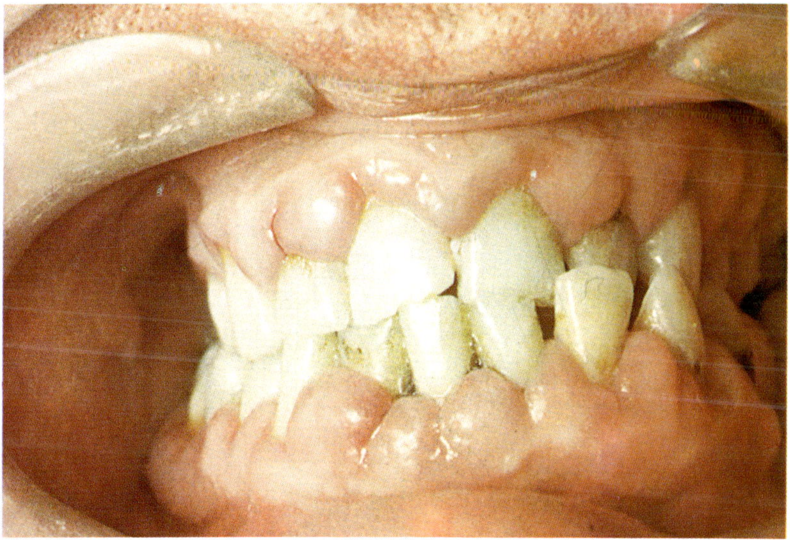

115

Fig. 122. In this case of severe chronic periodontitis with deep pocketing and bone loss there is, in addition, deposition of bismuth producing a blue-black discoloration of the gingival tissue. Such discoloration may also be due to lead or mercury. *(523.41; N.985.0)*

Fig. 123. Periodic neutropenia producing an intense gingivitis and inflammation of the whole oral mucosa. Deep penetrating fuso-spirochaetal ulceration may occur on the gingiva or unattached oral mucosa. A similar picture may be seen in leukaemia. *(288.X0)*

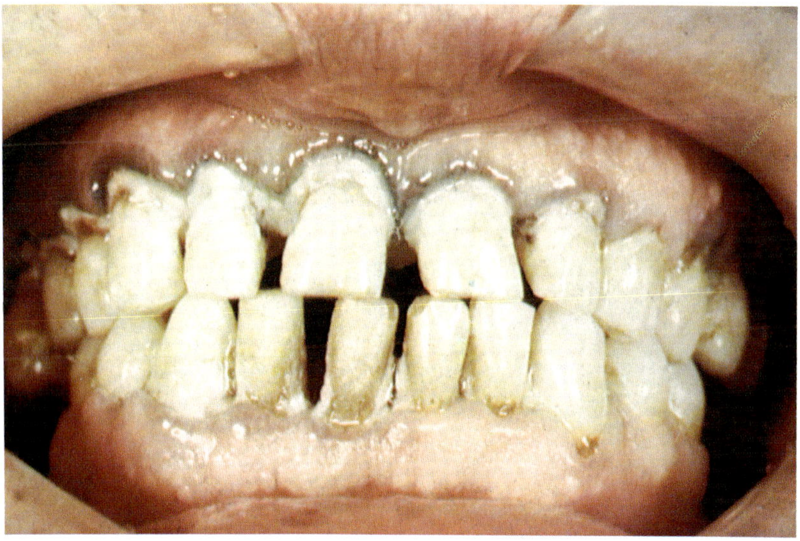

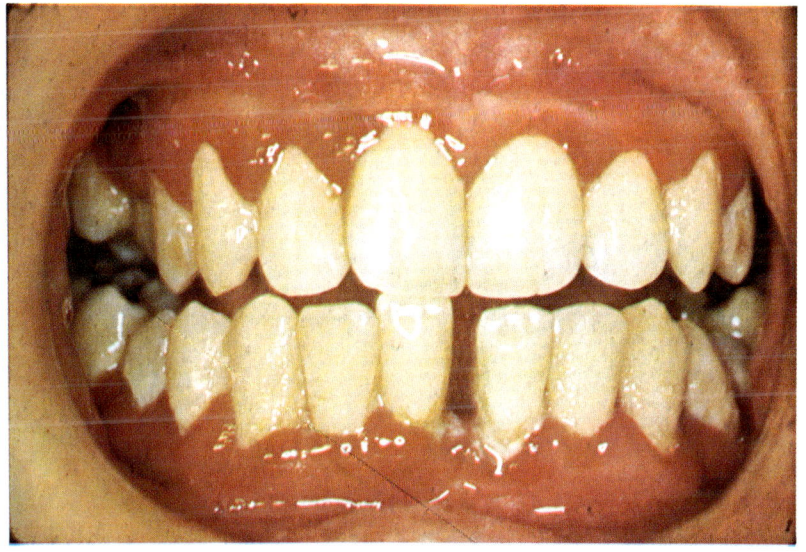

Fig. 124. Reticulum cell sarcoma of the gingiva, a very unusual condition. *(200.00)*

Fig. 125. The same case showing cervical metastases.

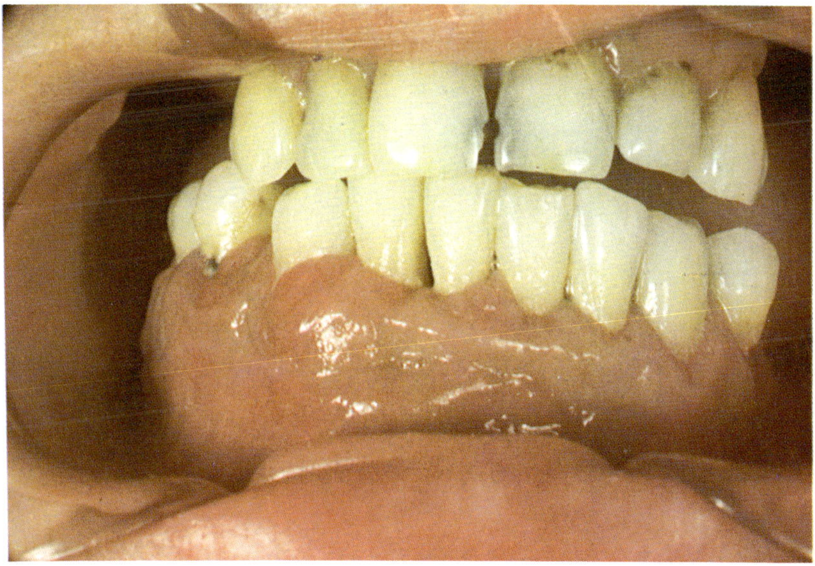

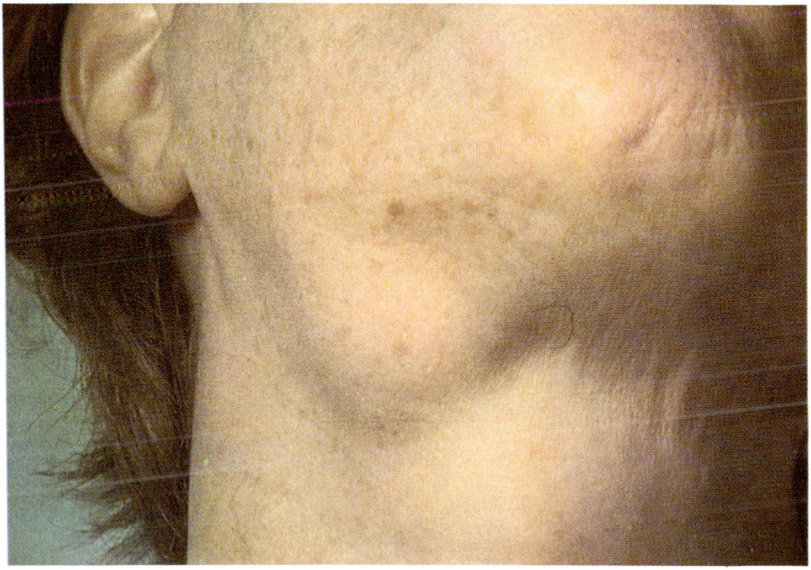

119

Fig. 126. A pyogenic granuloma of the gingival margin — a common site for the lesion. It grows rapidly and painlessly and bleeds freely. *(210.43)*

Fig. 127. Another pyogenic granuloma, here occurring in pregnancy, and often referred to colloquially as a "pregnancy tumour". Note the rather florid gingivitis with little radial vessels in the gingival margin typical of hormonal gingivitis. *(634.V1)*

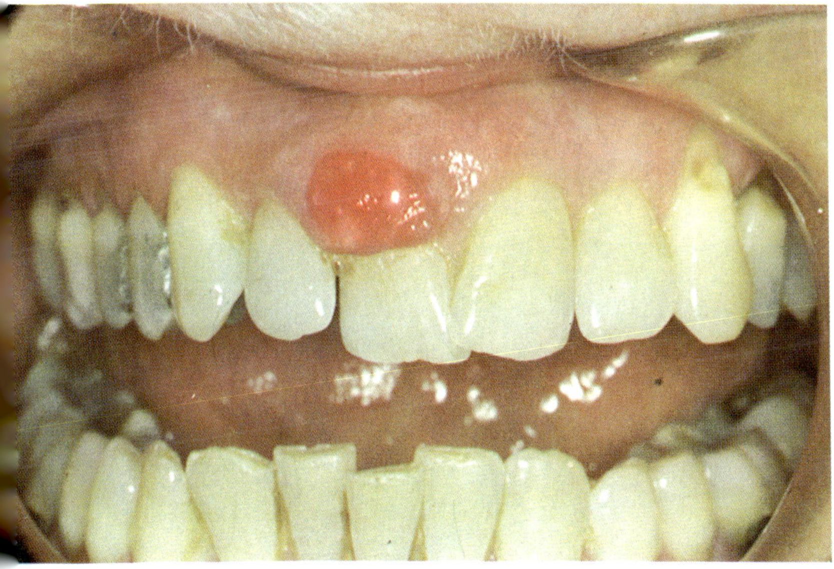

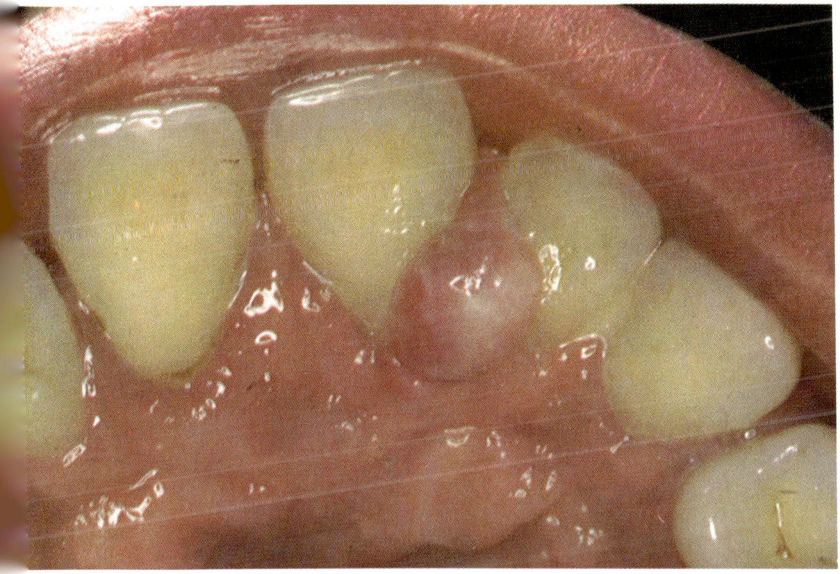

121

Fig. 128. A severe proliferative gingivitis, here associated with the malignant granuloma of the nose. A similar picture may occur in leukaemia (particularly monocytic) and scurvy. *(446.2X)*

Fig. 129. Giant-cell granuloma (peripheral) of the gingival tissue. Although extensive, this was attached by a pedicle distal to the lower right second premolar and only just involved underlying bone. Giant-cell granuloma of the jaws may be central or peripheral and is almost unique to the jaws. Identical lesions may occur, however, throughout the skeleton, including the jaws, in hyperparathyroidism, and this disorder must be excluded by estimation of the serum calcium. *(210.43)*

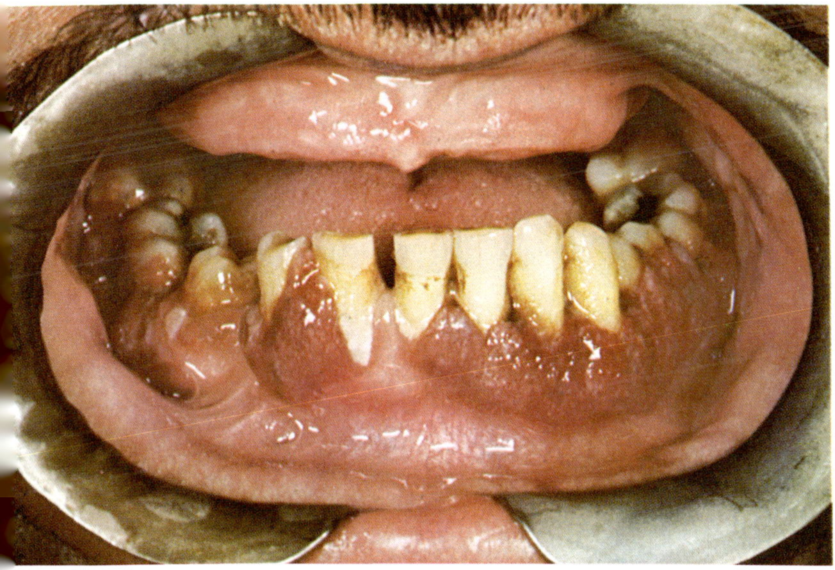

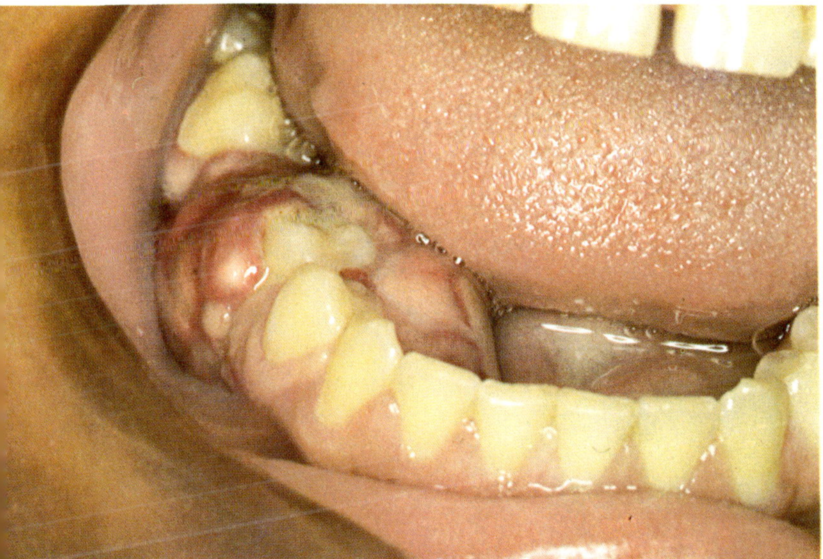

123

Fig. 130. These teeth, the upper right second and third molars, are fused together by cementum. The third molar is unerupted and the extraction of the second molar presents great problems. *(521.6X)*

Fig. 131. A neonate with a "natal" tooth. These teeth are predeciduous and can be removed easily because they have no roots. *(520.60)*

Fig. 132. Another neonate with a smooth pedunculated swelling of the lower gum pad. It is a myoblastoma or congenital epulis. *(210.43)*

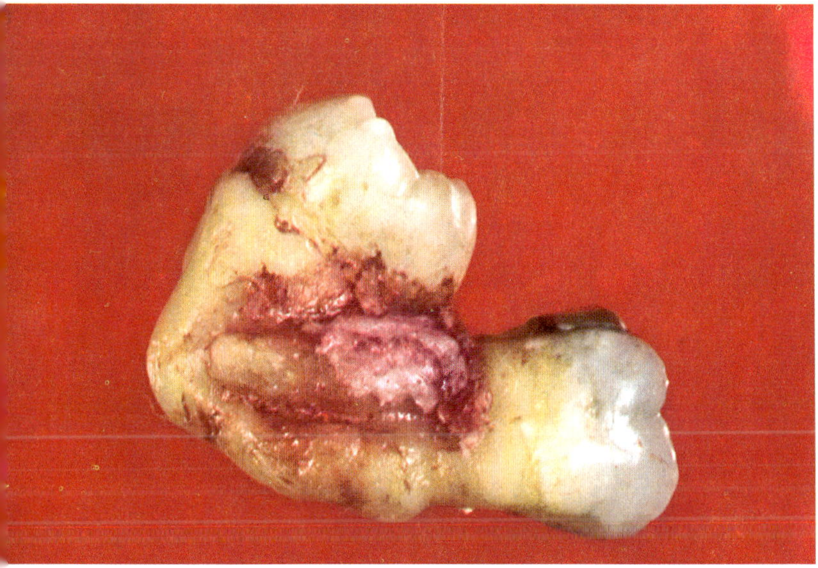

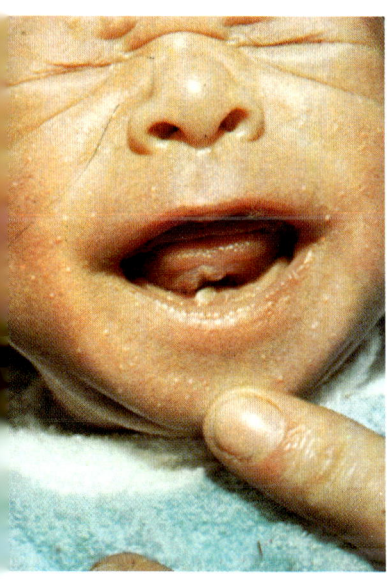
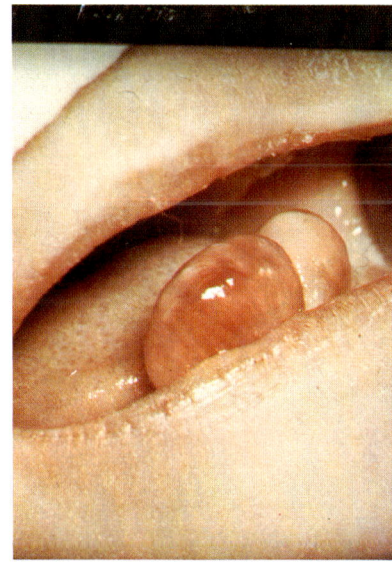

SECTION FIVE: **THE "LUMPS"**

Fig. 133. A fibro-epithelial polyp attached just inside the commissure of the mouth. The lesion is soft and the surface is partly hyperkeratinised — due to excessive friction. *(528.90)*

Fig. 134. Another fibro-epithelial polyp of the lip, but here the surface is tessellated by extensive hyperkeratosis and is very similar to a papilloma. *(528.90)*

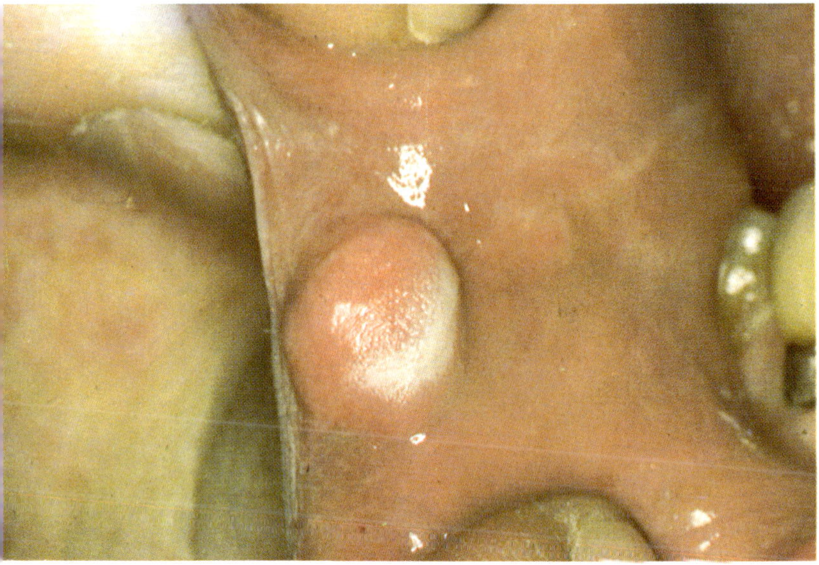

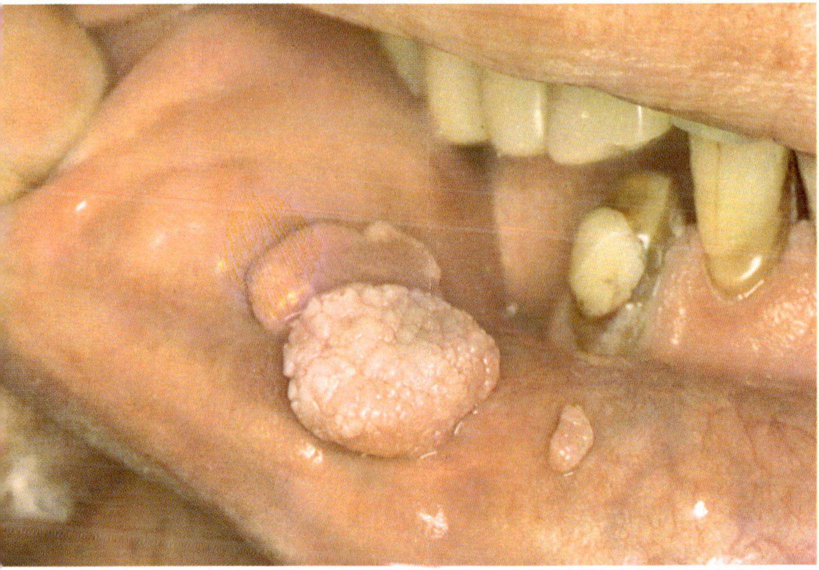

Fig. 135. Extensive traumatic fibro-epithelial hyperplasia of the upper labial sulcus (denture granuloma). This situation is inimical to successful denture support. *(528.90)*

Fig. 136. This patient had a well established oro-antral fistula through which an antral polyp had prolapsed and caused the patient considerable alarm. Such a transparent structure with clear fluid contents appears blue by reflected light on a dark background, *i.e.* when in the antrum. When in the mouth its true nature is revealed as it is viewed by transmitted light. The contents are pale yellow, and delicate vessels course in the wall. *(N998.60)*

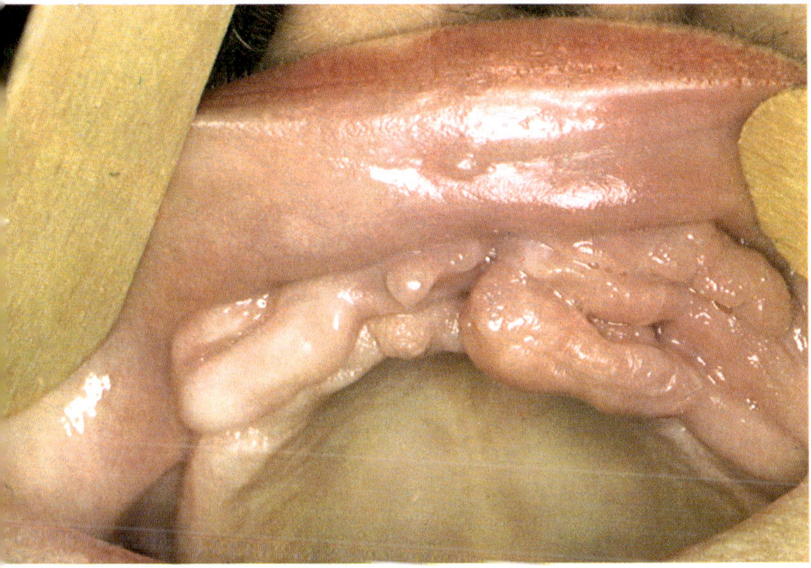

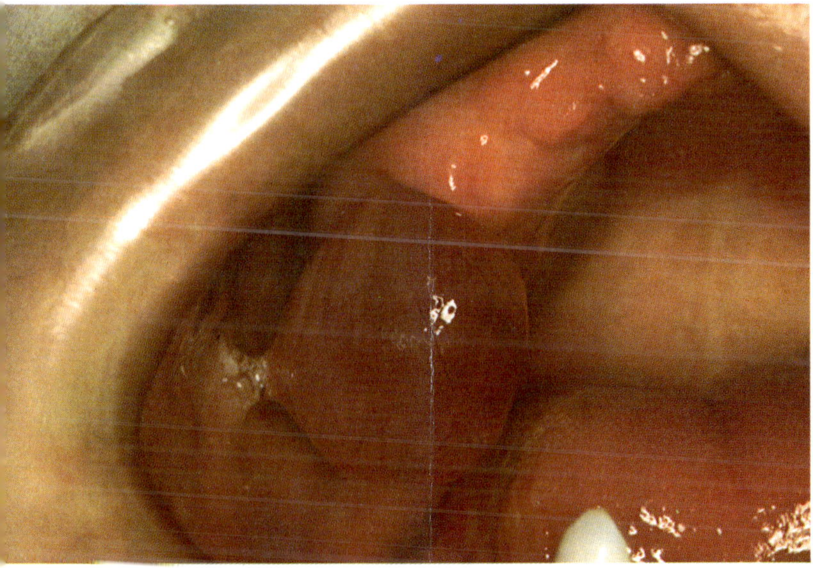

Fig. 137. A large giant-cell granuloma of the upper alveolus in an ill-kept mouth. The colour is rather paler than is usual. *(210.43)*

Fig. 138. A true fibroma of the alveolus. Note that its colour is pale; the lesion was firm to the touch. It grew progressively and was encapsulated. Benign tumours are rare in the mouth, as distinct from the common fibro-epithelial polyp. *(210.43)*

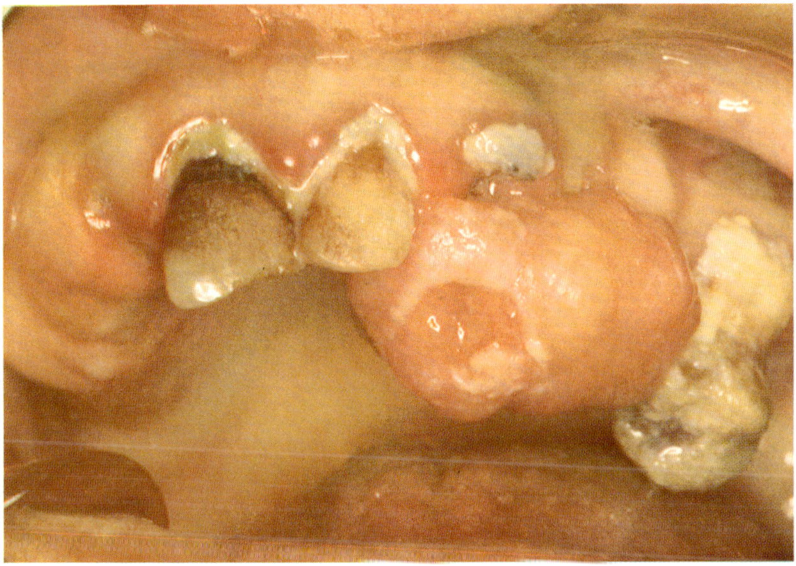

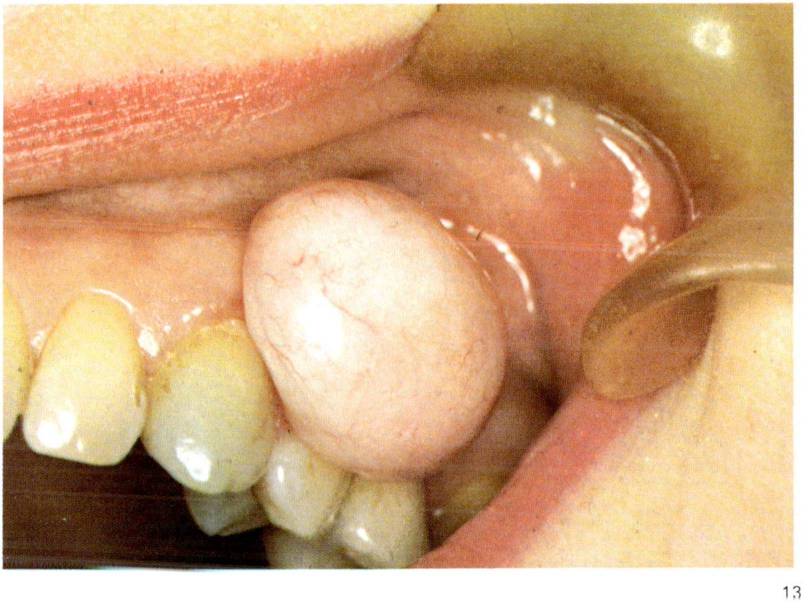

Fig. 139. These small white raised nodules are epidermoid cysts lying just beneath the epithelium. They are frequently present in the newborn when they are termed Epstein's pearls. *(528.40)*

Fig. 140. Here there is a raised white lesion of the right alveolus; there is also expansion of the alveolar bone buccally and palatally. This is an odontogenic keratocyst (epidermoid) which has ruptured buccally and is discharging its cheesy contents. *(522.82)*

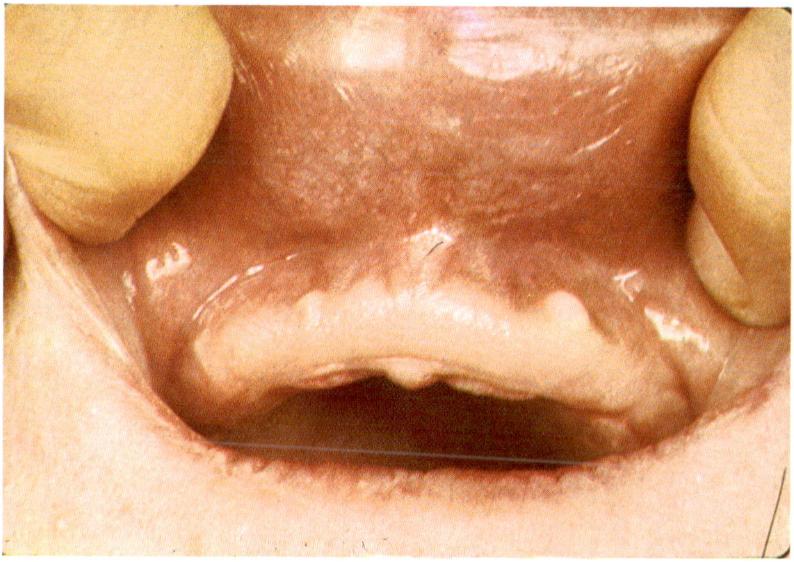

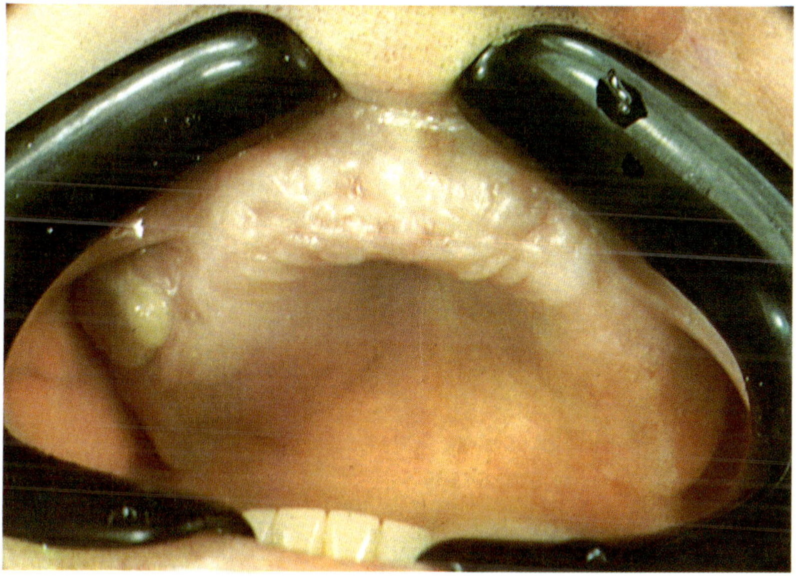

133

Fig. 141. Another example of herniation of an antral polyp into the mouth via an oro-antral fistula. In this case haemorrhage into the polyp had occurred. *(N998.60)*

Fig. 142. Chronic periapical suppuration around the left maxillary second incisor which is associated with sinus formation. The resemblance to a fibro-epithelial polyp is striking. *(522.7X)*

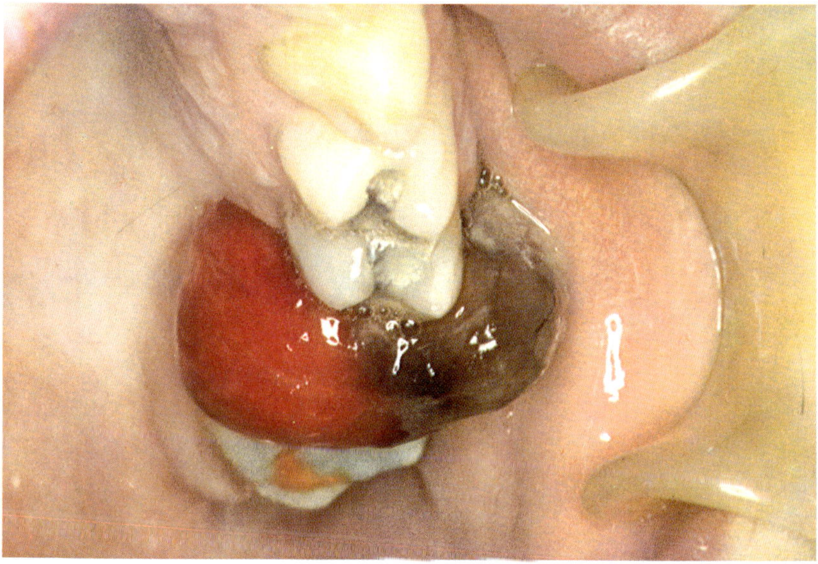

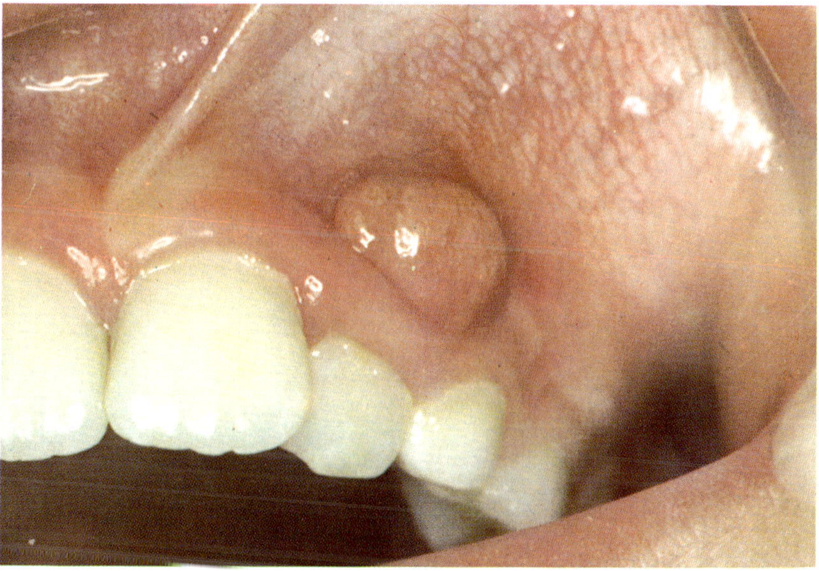

135

Fig. 143. A dental cyst of radicular origin on the upper right lateral incisor. Note the typical buccal expansion with bluish coloration where the cyst has destroyed the buccal plate. Displacement of the upper right canine is also evident. *(522.80)*

Fig. 144. Standard occlusal x-ray of the case above showing the well-defined radiolucency centred above the upper second incisor. The thin shell of expanded buccal plate is also clearly demonstrable.

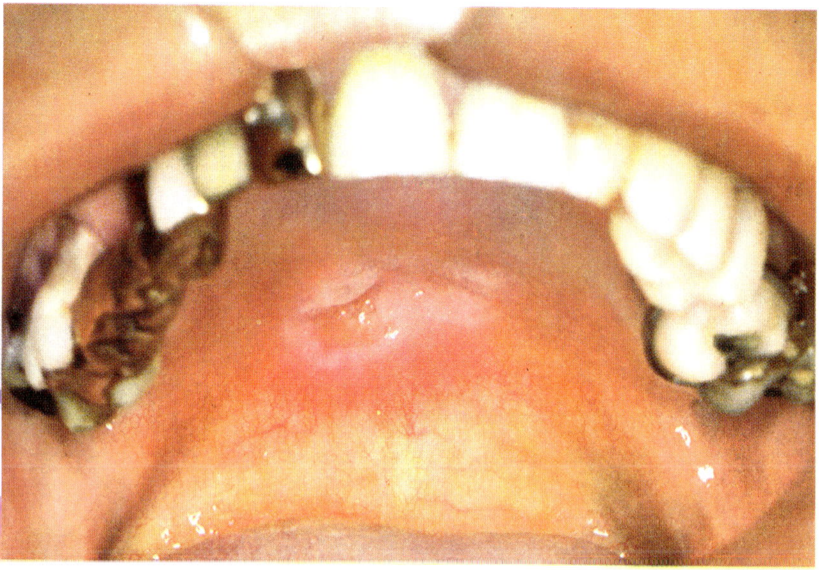

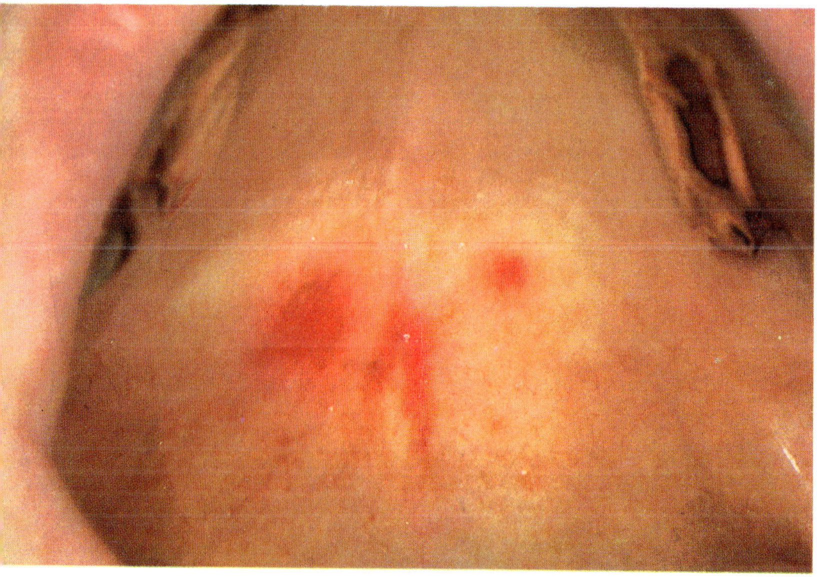

181

Fig. 189. This black lesion, looking like caviar spread on the palate, is a malignant melanoma. *(172.3X)*

Fig. 190. Melanoma of the oral cavity has to be distinguished from racial pigmentation of the alveolar mucosa and amalgam tattoo. The latter has a more pronounced blue-grey coloration. *(757.10)*

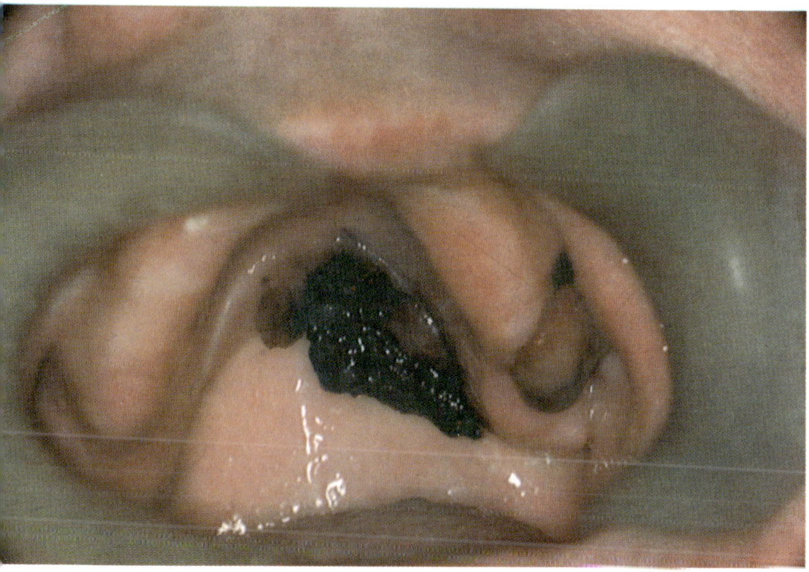

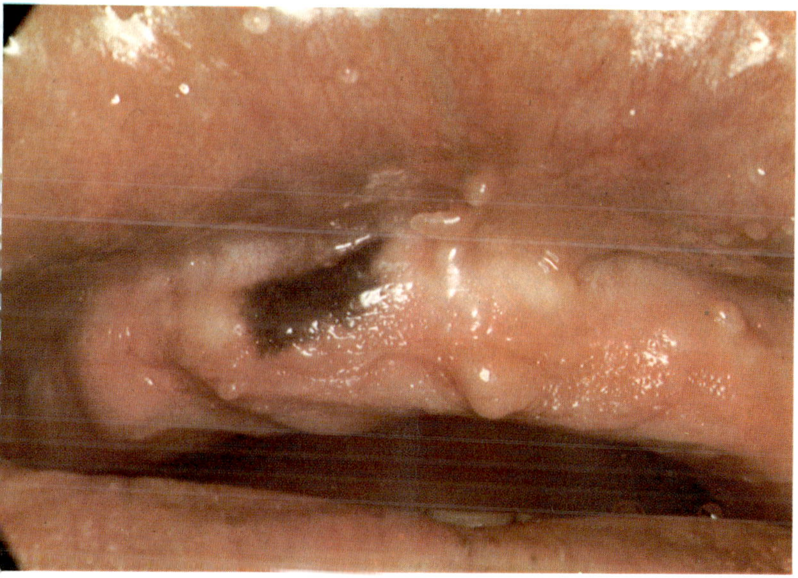

183

Fig. 191. An odontogenic keratocyst of the upper right jaw with considerable palatal expansion. Unlike simple dental cysts, this lesion may expand rapidly and it shows a marked tendency to recur following treatment. *(526.01)*

Fig. 192. This small, tense bluish swelling above the upper right lateral incisor might have been a dental cyst, but the tooth was vital and no bone destruction was apparent on x-ray. The cyst lay between the alveolar bone and overlying mucoperiosteum. It is developmental in origin and akin to the higher nasolabial cyst. *(526.18)*

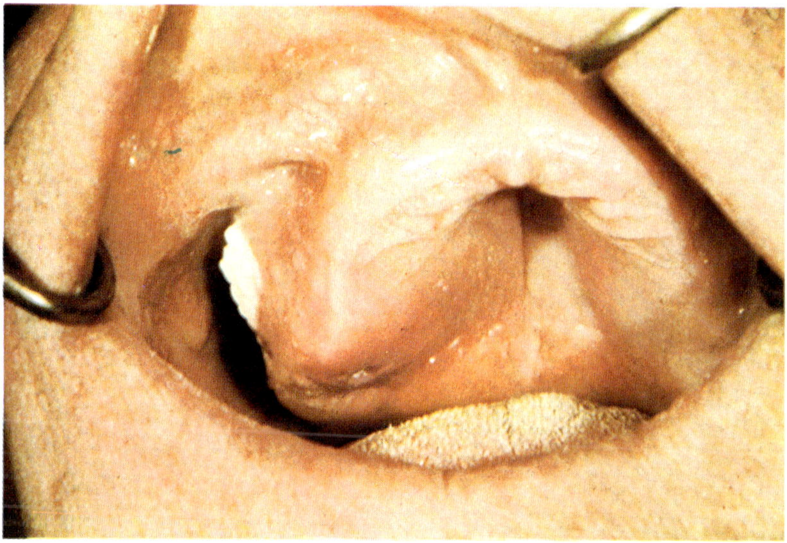

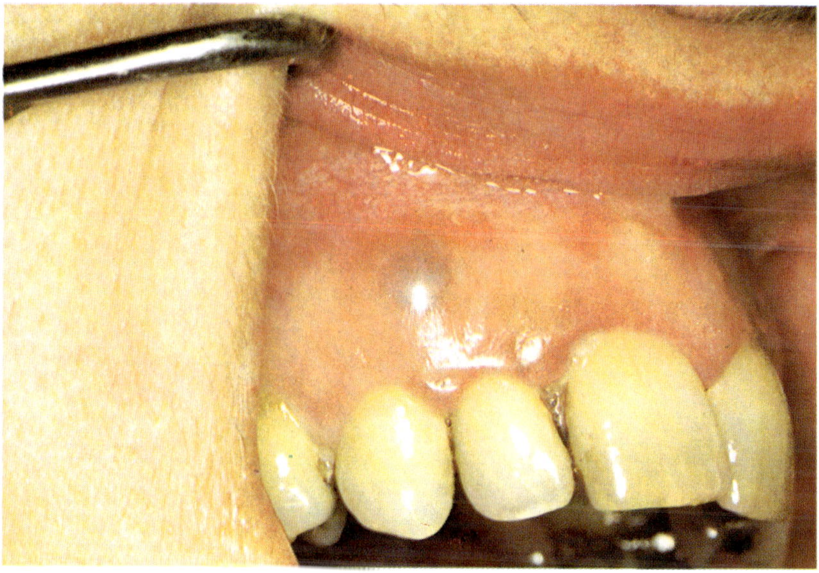

185

Figs. 193 & 194. This patient has some upward displacement of the left eye associated with infra-orbital anaesthesia. Intra-orally there is buccal expansion of the upper alveolus. This is an advanced squamous cell carcinoma of the antrum. A malignancy of this type is the commonest neoplasm found in the maxillary sinus. *(160.2X)*

Figs. 195 & 196. Another antral carcinoma, here with considerable facial swelling. The x-ray shows the opacity of the right antrum and extensive bone destruction of its superior and lateral bony walls. Malignant tumours of the maxillary sinus may also encroach on the orbit, nose and infratemporal fossa, and if these structures are involved by direct spread, typical signs and symptoms are produced. *(160.2X)*

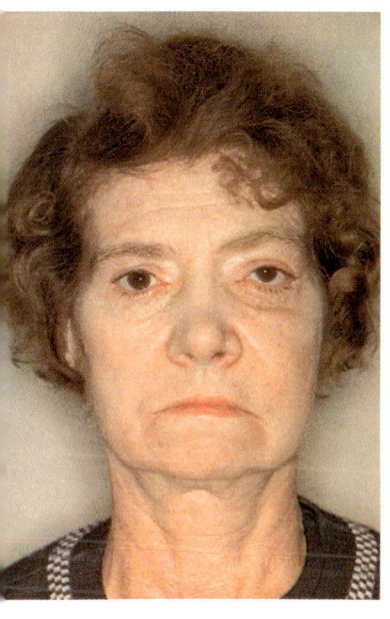
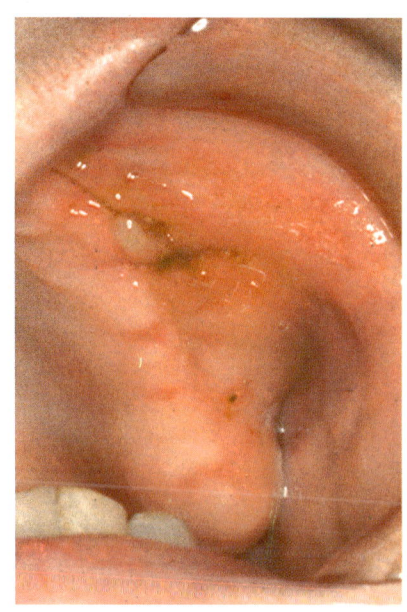
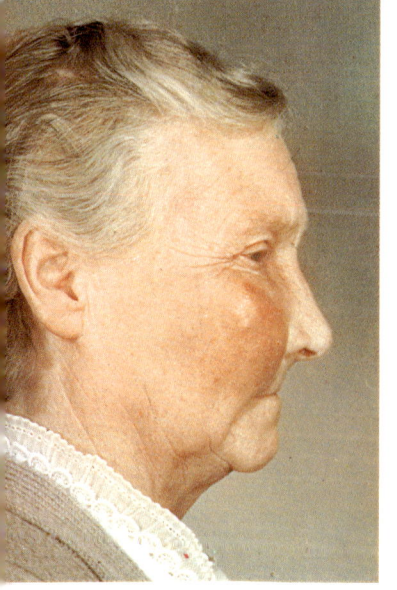
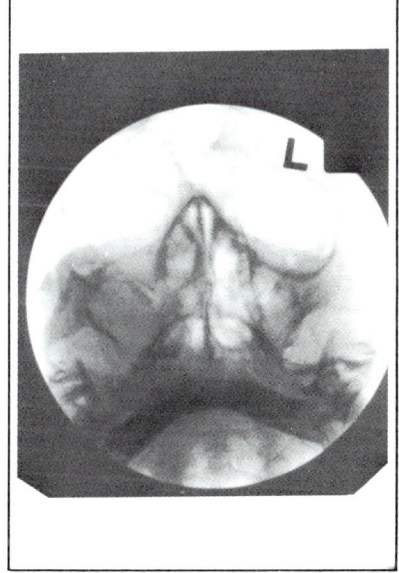

187

SECTION EIGHT: **THE TONGUE**

Fig. 197. Tongue-tie, due to an abnormally short lingual fraenum. This causes no disability and such patients are frequently seen in the second decade. *(750.01)*

Fig. 198. A crenated tongue is usually of no significance, but it might be indicative of macroglossia. *(529.90)*

Figs. 199 & 200. "Geographical" tongue—erythema migrans linguae. As can be seen, it is simply a depapillated patch of the dorsum from which the filiform papillae have disappeared but the fungiform remain. The second picture **(fig. 200)** indicates a typical distribution of this common and usually asymptomatic lesion. A characteristic feature is the alteration in the configuration of the smooth red areas, the sudden healing and then reappearance in another part of the tongue (hence "migrans"). *(529.1X)*

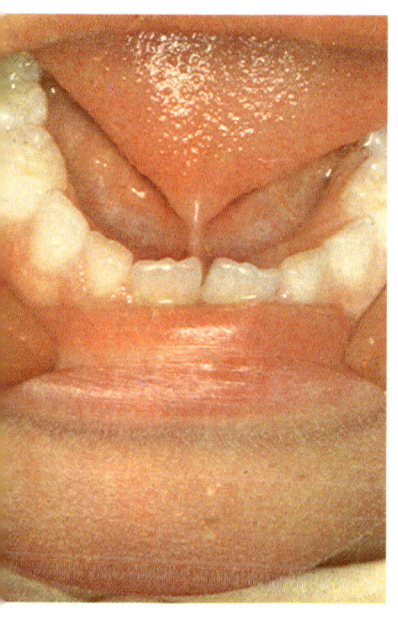
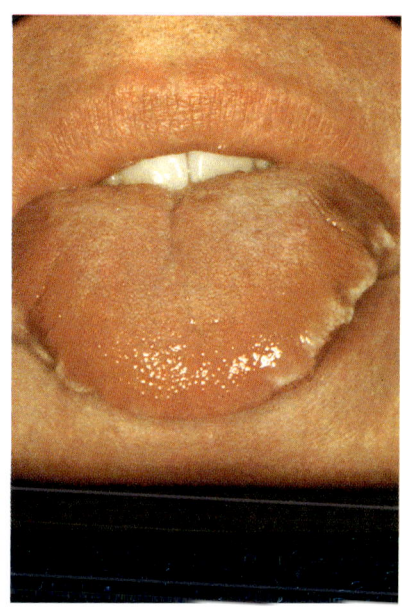
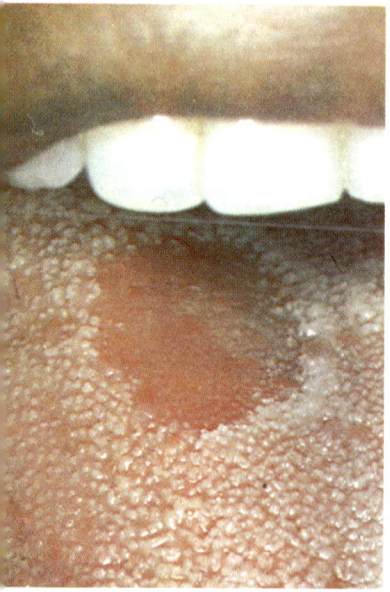
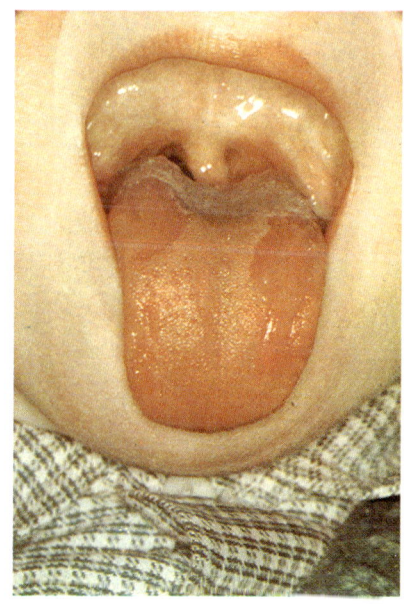

Fig. 201. Black hairy tongue is of unknown aetiology, but black or brown-black staining of the tongue may complicate the local use in the mouth of concentrated hydrogen peroxide solutions and topical antibiotics. Liquid iron preparations taken habitually may also cause the mid-dorsal area of the tongue to acquire a dense black discoloration. *(529.31)*

Fig. 202. The brown discoloration typically associated with the administration of antibiotics. *(N.960)*

Fig. 203. A mucous patch of the tongue – a lesion of secondary syphilis. *(091.20)*

Fig. 204. The tongue of tertiary syphilis with fissuring and hyperkeratosis. *(095.X2)*

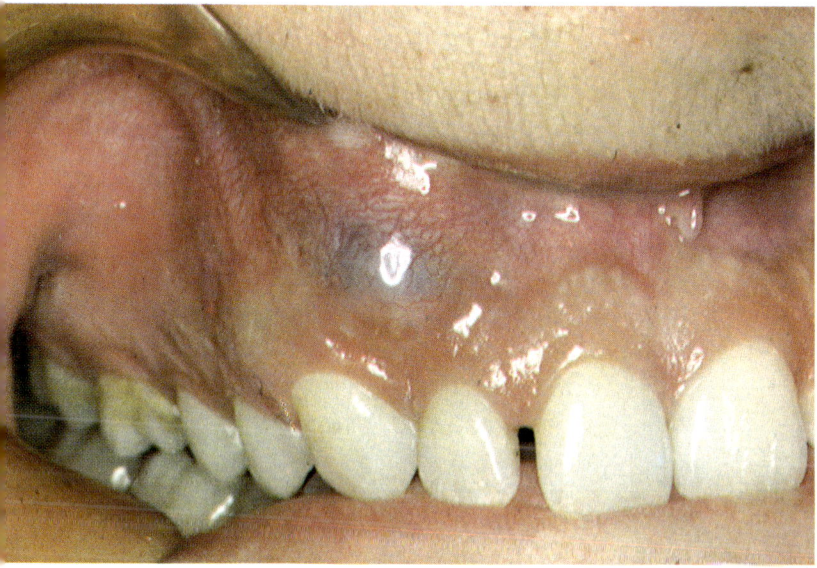

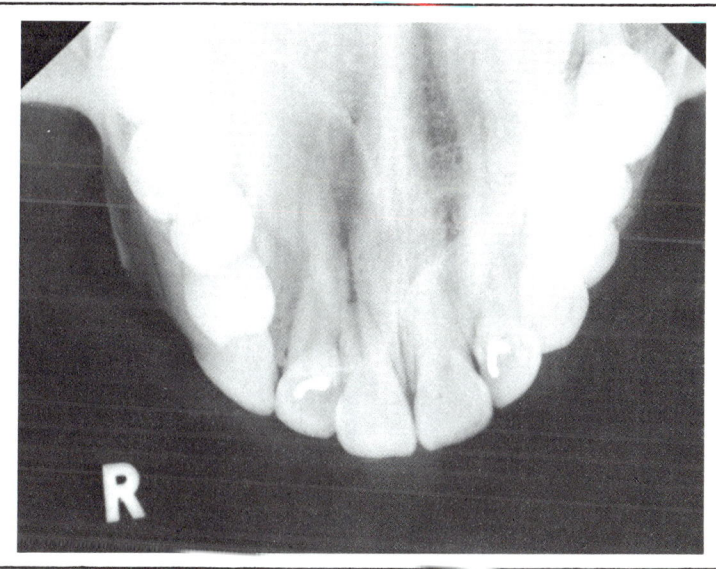

Fig. 145. Expansion of the upper alveolus, in this case bony hard and with normally coloured overlying mucosa. This is an exostosis or "osteoma". *(213.X0)*

Fig. 146. The x-ray shows the pedunculated nature of the lesion and the rather dense bone comprising its substance.

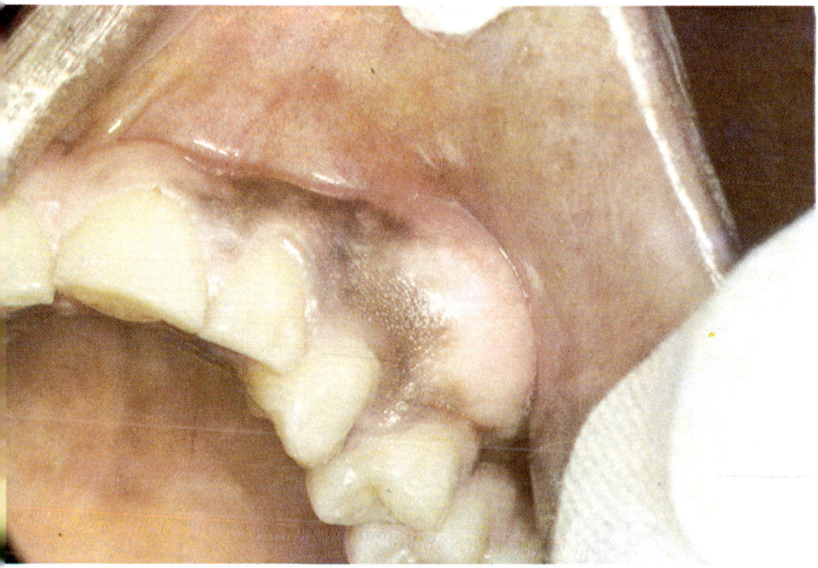

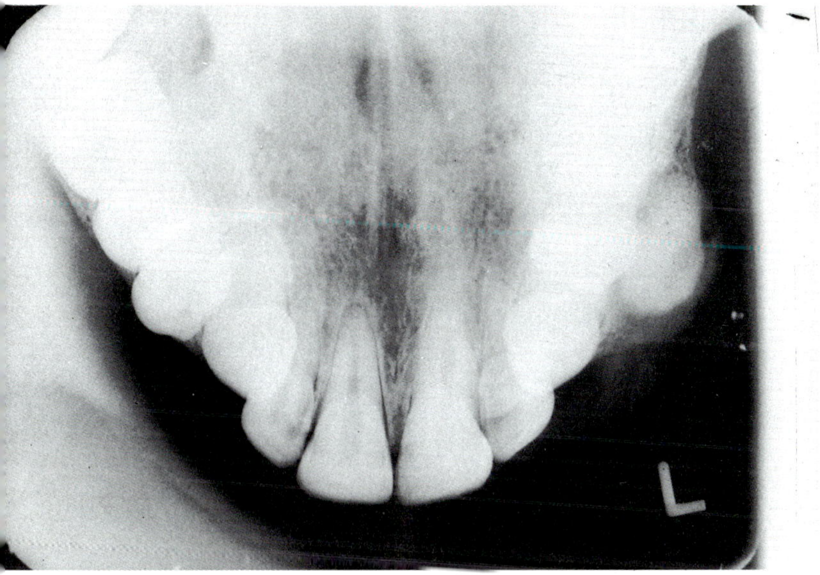

139

Fig. 147. A further example of a peripheral giant-cell granuloma of the upper alveolus, a lesion which may eventually cause divarication of adjacent teeth and pressure resorption of the immediate underlying bone. A large granuloma may become ulcerated if repeatedly bitten by opposing teeth and, rarely, interference with mastication may be experienced. *(210.43)*

Fig. 148. A large pyogenic granuloma of the upper incisor region in a young child. *(210.43)*

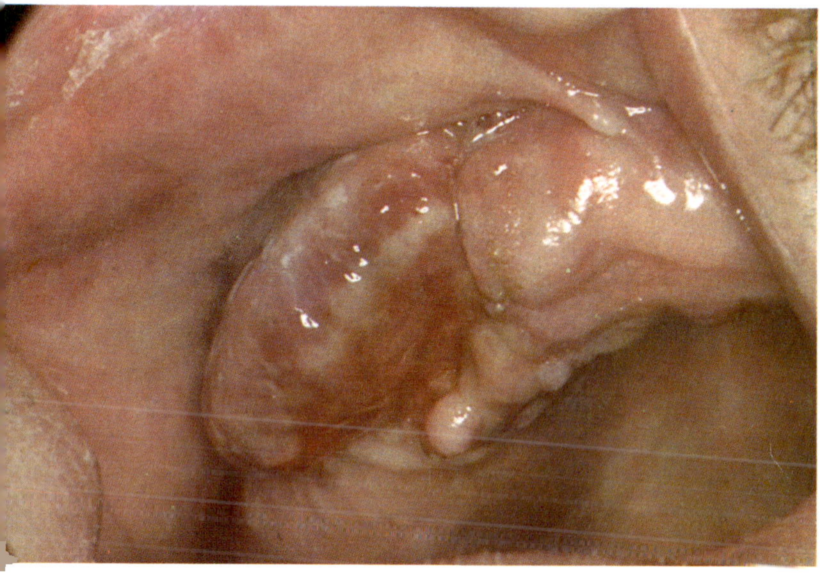

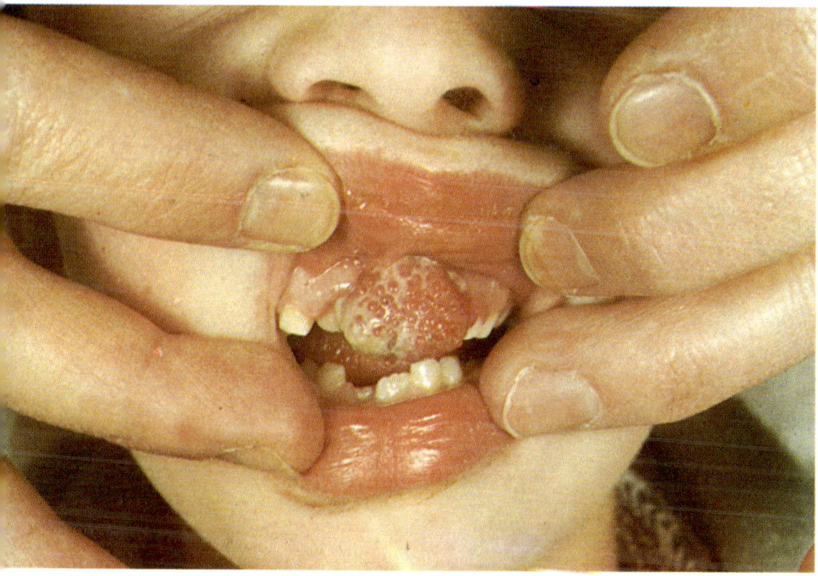

141

Fig. 149. A large but superficial squamous cell carcinoma involving most of the right hard palate and alveolar ridge and, in part, the soft palate. *(145.10)*

Fig. 150. Yet another prolapsed antral polyp. This, with **figs. 137** and **142,** illustrates the variations in the clinical features of one condition. This polypus is quite granulomatous in appearance. *(N998.60)*

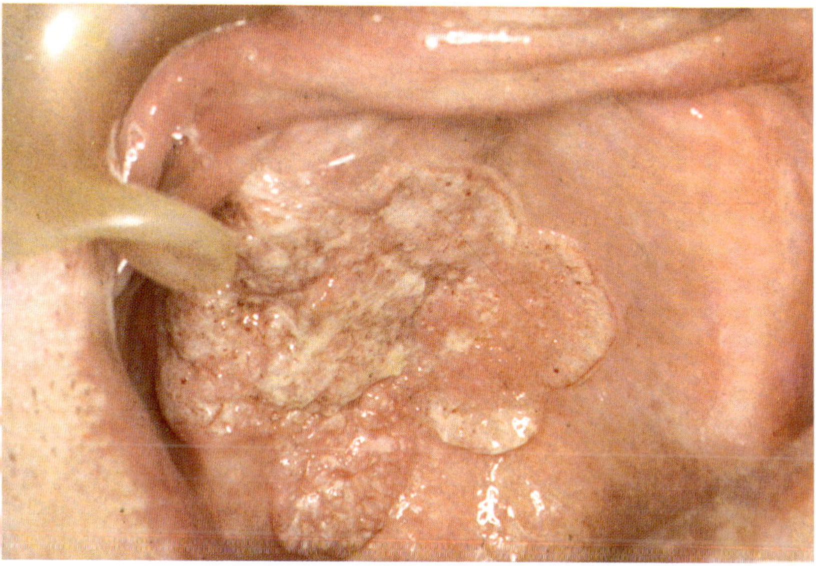

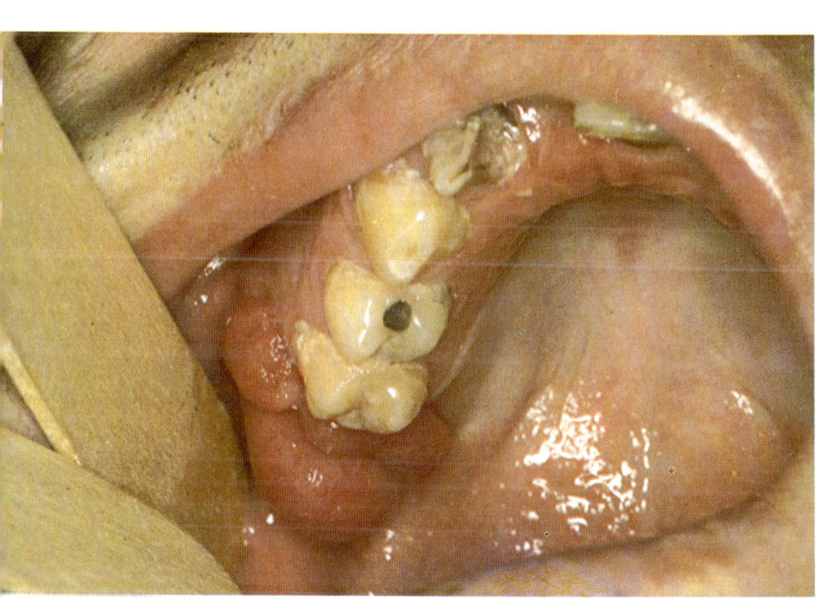

143

Fig. 151. An extensive squamous cell carcinoma of the hard palate with a papilliferous surface typical of most oral carcinomas. *(145.10)*

Fig. 152. The carcinoma in **fig. 151** arose beneath a denture with a suction disc which had been worn for many years. The irritation produced by this denture may have been partly responsible for the development of the neoplasm.

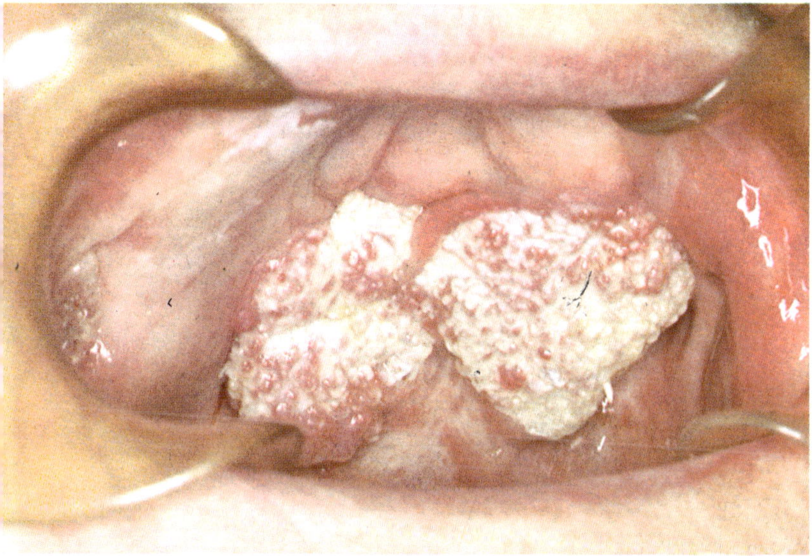

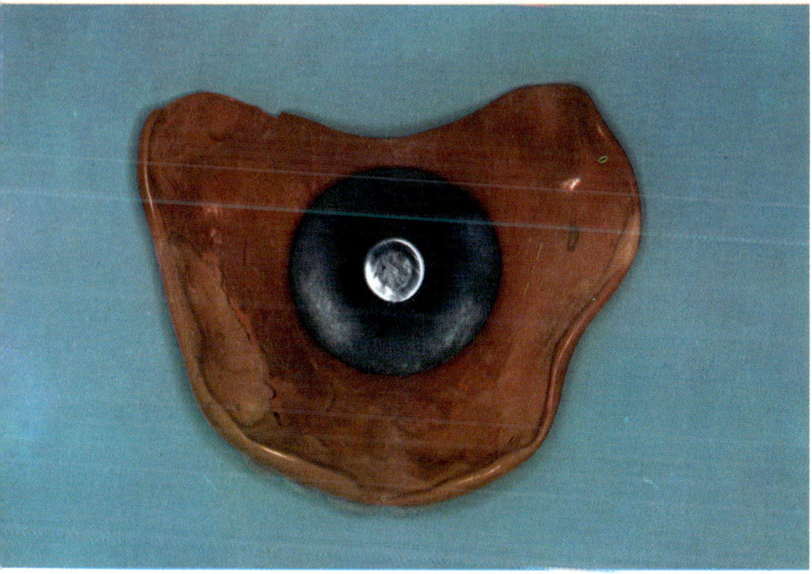

145

Fig. 153. A nodular mass on the upper alveolus which might have been a carcinoma but which was, in fact, an amelanotic melanoma. *(172.3X)*

Fig. 154. This view of the patient's neck reveals metastatic deposits from the tumour in the regional (submandibular) lymph nodes.

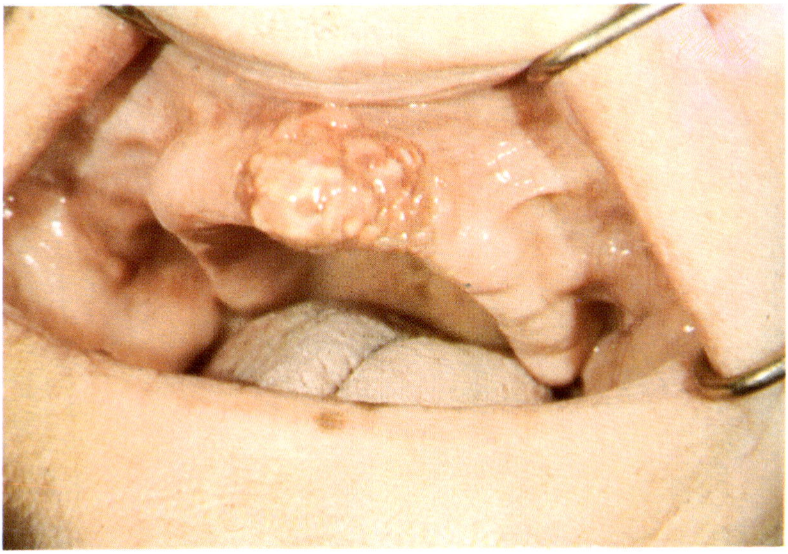

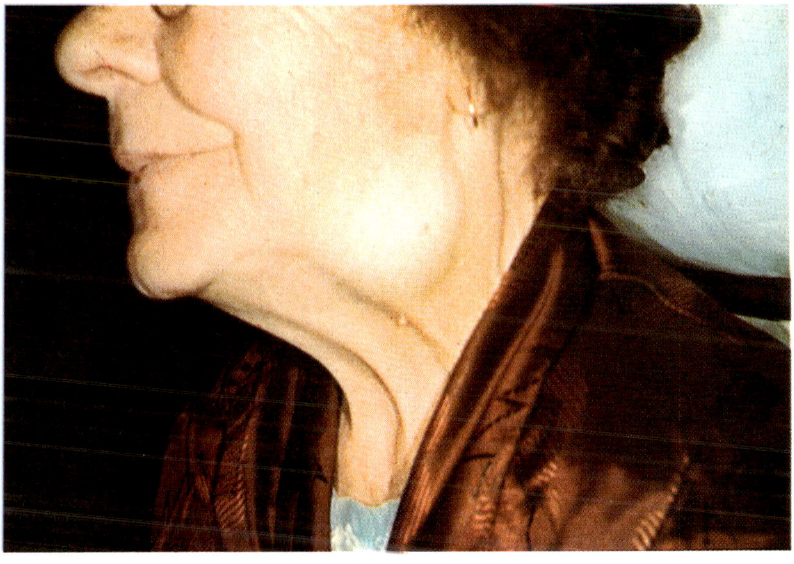

147

Fig. 155. An ulcerated area with a nodular reddened edge on the upper alveolus which proved to be an angiosarcoma. Metastases were already present when the patient was first seen. *(171.0X)*

Fig. 156. A lesion similar (in appearance) to the former, but due to trauma of the upper ridge by a lower molar tooth during an alcoholic stupor. The ulcer had recurred several times in the preceding year but remitted on removal of the causative lower tooth. *(N910.0X)*

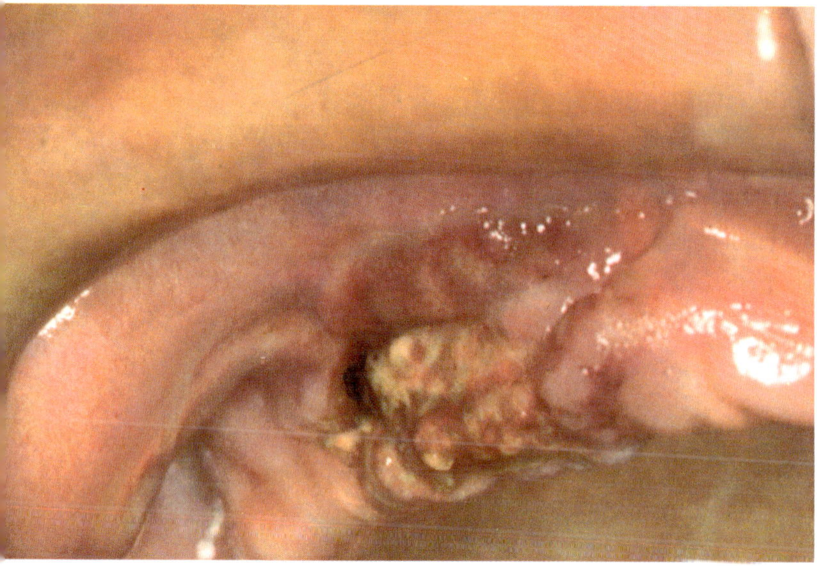

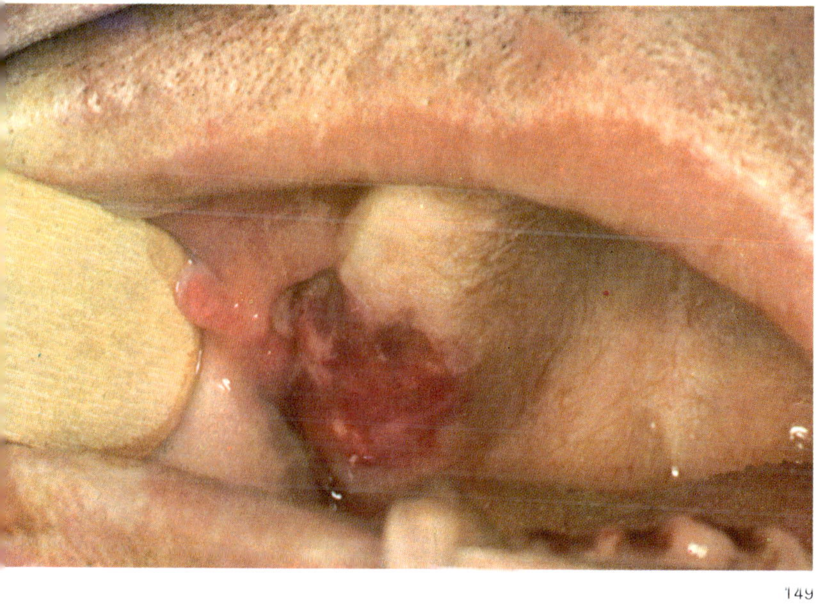

149

Fig. 157. A small area of fibro-epithelial hyperplasia due to irritation of the posterior end of an upper partial denture. *(528.90)*

Fig. 158. Adenocarcinoma of the hard palate. In addition to the considerable submucosal swelling at this site, ulceration is present typical of malignant "salivary" gland tumours. *(142.82)*

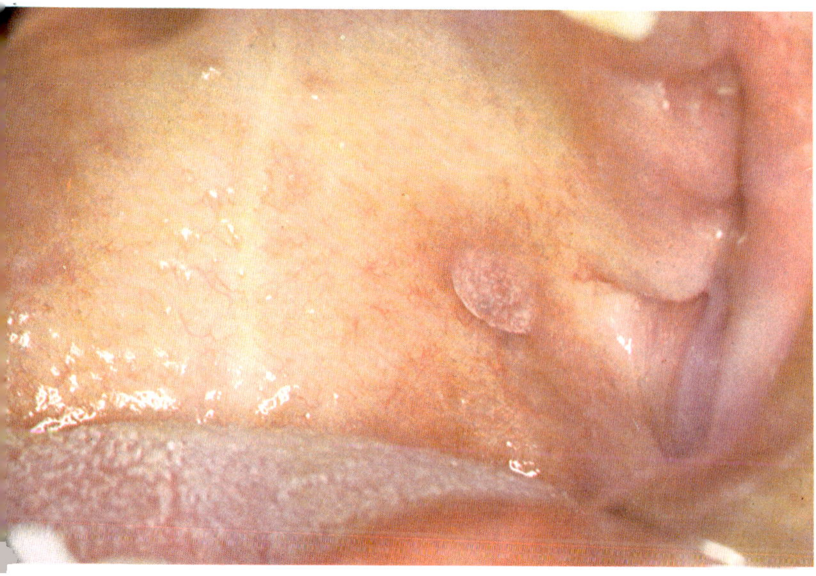

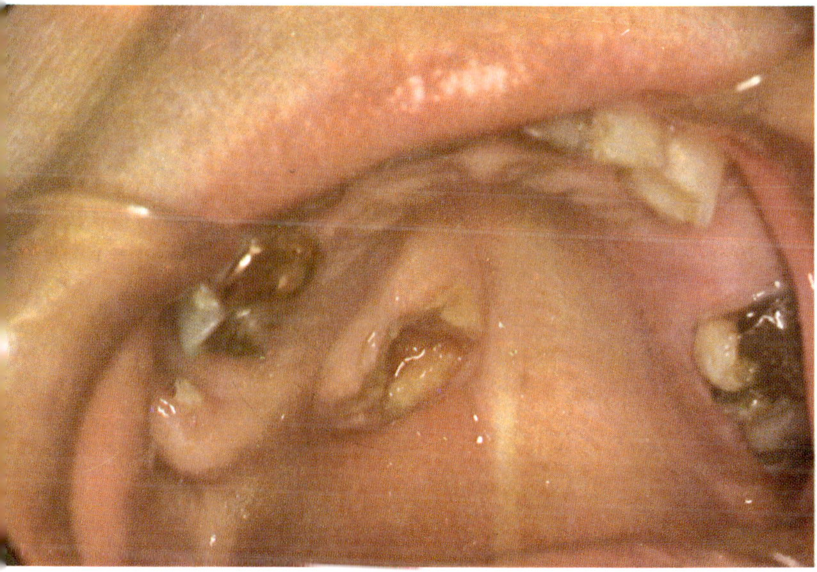

Fig. 159. Pleomorphic adenoma of the hard/soft palate junction which is the commonest site of this tumour in the mouth. The surface is smooth or faintly lobulated and the overlying mucosa normal. *(210.23)*

Fig. 160. Here there is some expansion of the alveolus with punched-out ulceration. X-ray revealed diffuse bone destruction, and biopsy established the diagnosis of multiple myelomatosis. *(203.X0)*

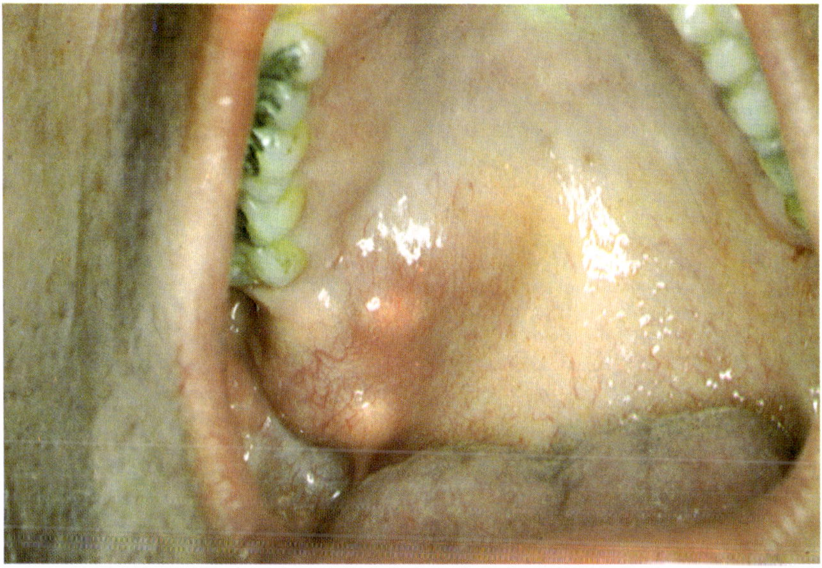

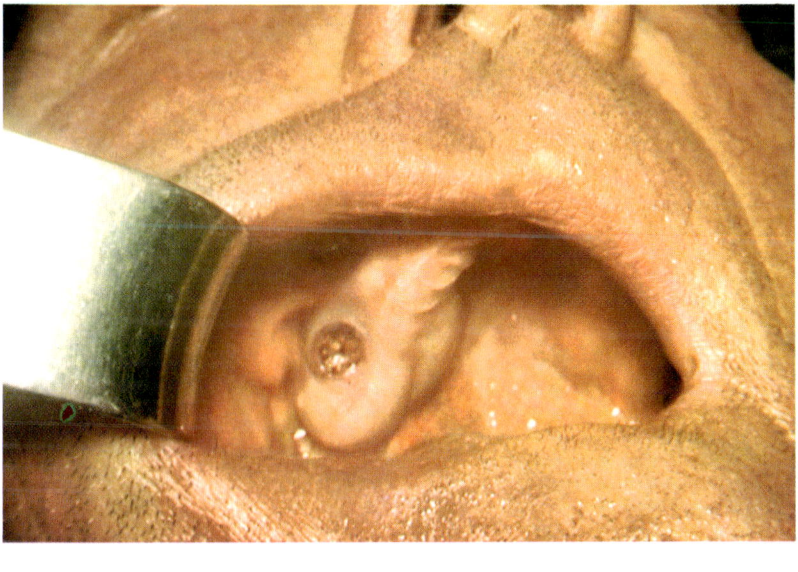

153

Fig. 161. This ulcer of the upper alveolus developed slowly and its floor is of necrotic bone. The patient had previously received radiotherapy to the face and osteoradionecrosis was diagnosed. *(526.90)*

Fig. 162. Gross expansion of the left maxilla which was slowly progressive, producing facial deformity. The teeth are undisplaced, the mucosa normal and the swelling bony hard. X-ray and subsequent operation confirmed the diagnosis of fibrous dysplasia. *(526.95)*

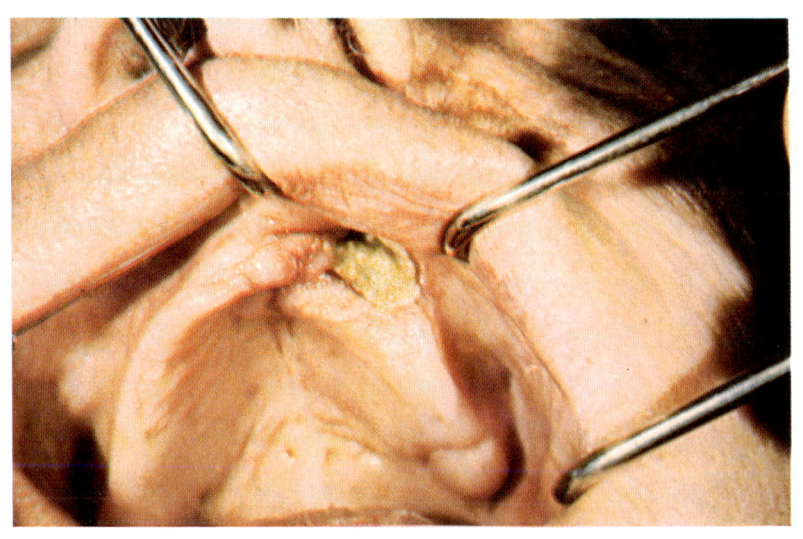
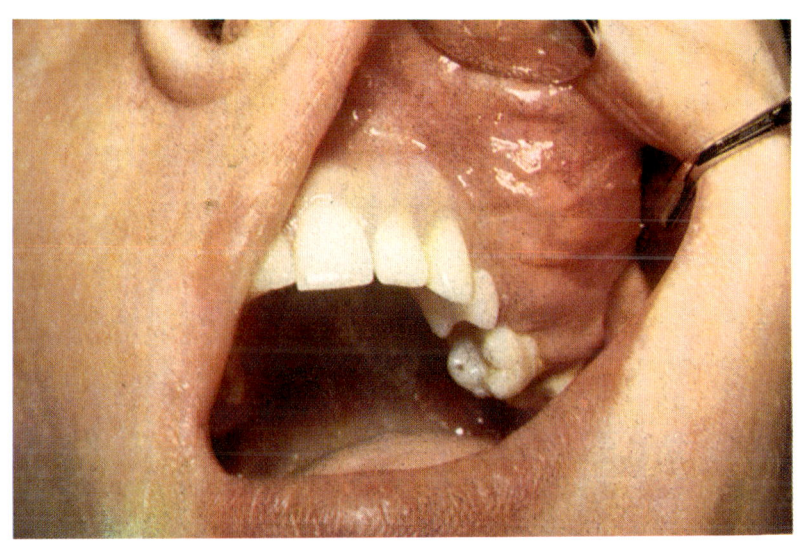

Fig. 163. This massive ulcerated neoplasm developed rapidly and was proved to be an anaplastic sarcoma. It arose in the region of the root of the soft palate. *(171.0X)*

Fig. 164. A massive intra-osseous lympho-reticular sarcoma of the left maxilla typical of Burkitt's lymphoma—soft tissue lesions also occur in abdominal organs, but lymph nodes are spared. *(202.20)*

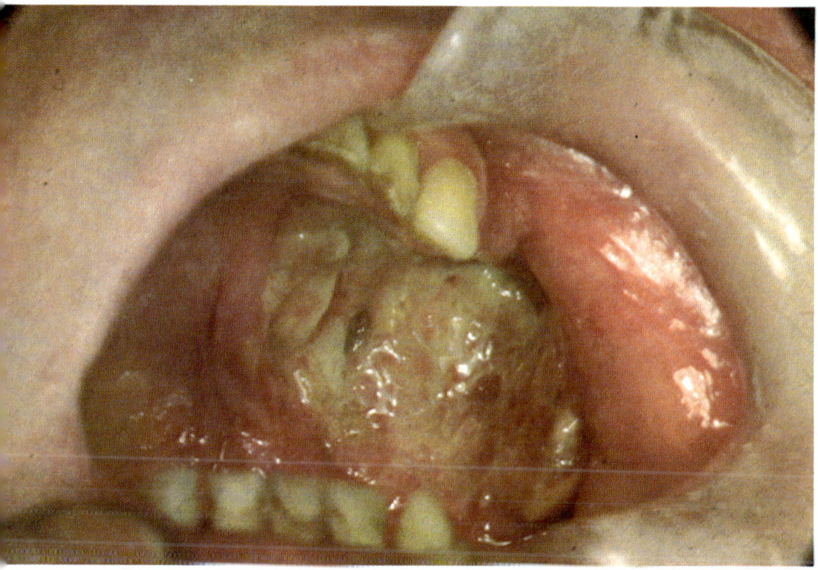

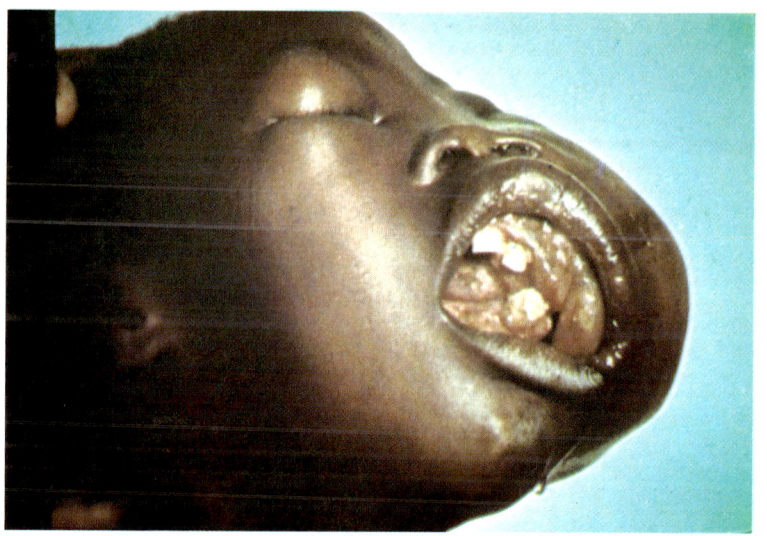

Fig. 165. A massive proliferative squamous cell carcinoma of the floor of the mouth invading the mandible. Oral carcinomas produce very few symptoms until quite large, and so only present late. The appearance is quite characteristic, but, in addition, the induration of the tissues is striking. *(144.XX)*

Fig. 166. This lesion grew rapidly out of a tooth-socket, and x-ray revealed localised bone destruction. The patient had an adenocarcinoma of the oesophago-gastric junction and this is a metastasis. It is possible that this secondary was not blood-borne, but became "seeded" in the socket from regurgitated malignant cells. *(197.90)*

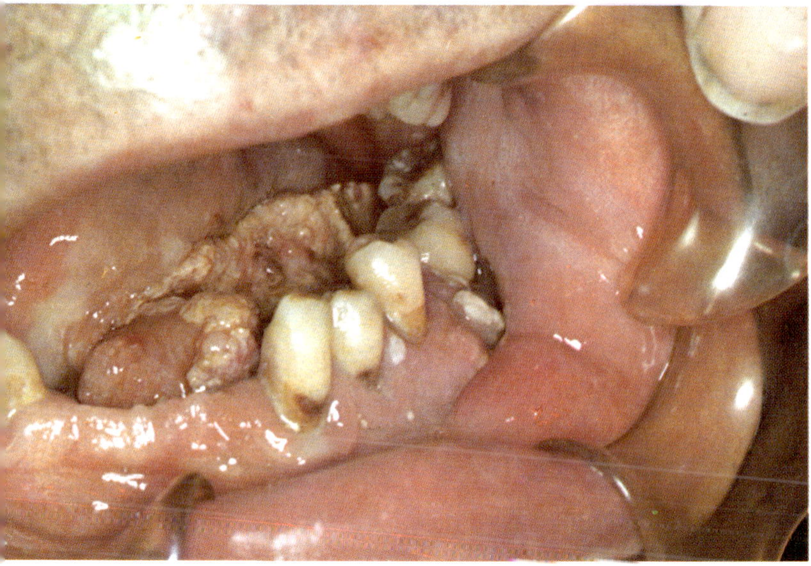

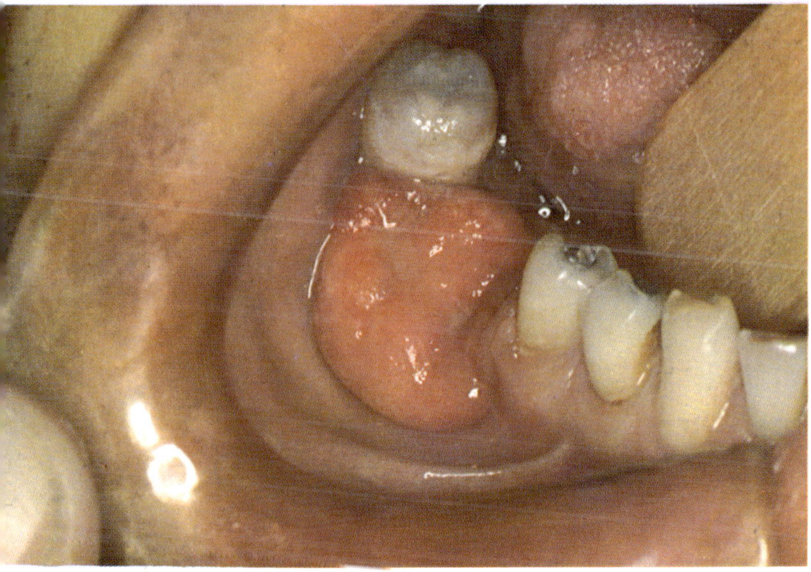

Fig. 167. A small nodular lesion of the floor of the mouth which proved to be a squamous cell carcinoma. Any small white, red or fissured lesion that is indurated, and for which there is no obvious cause, must be assumed to be a carcinoma, and biopsy is essential. *(144.XX)*

Fig. 168. Pleomorphic adenoma of the floor of the mouth derived from the sublingual salivary gland. *(210.22)*

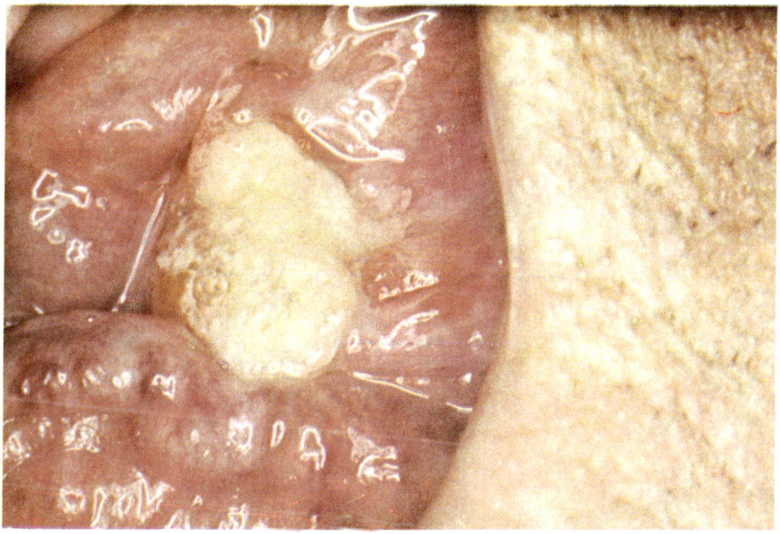

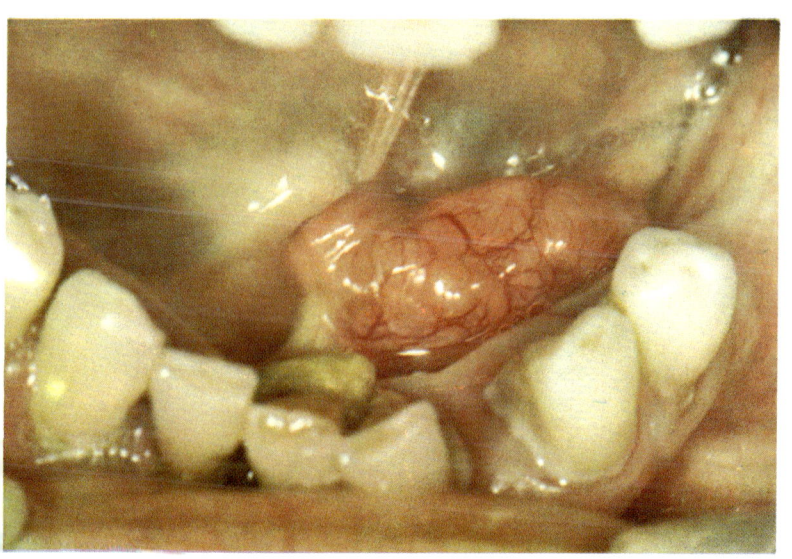

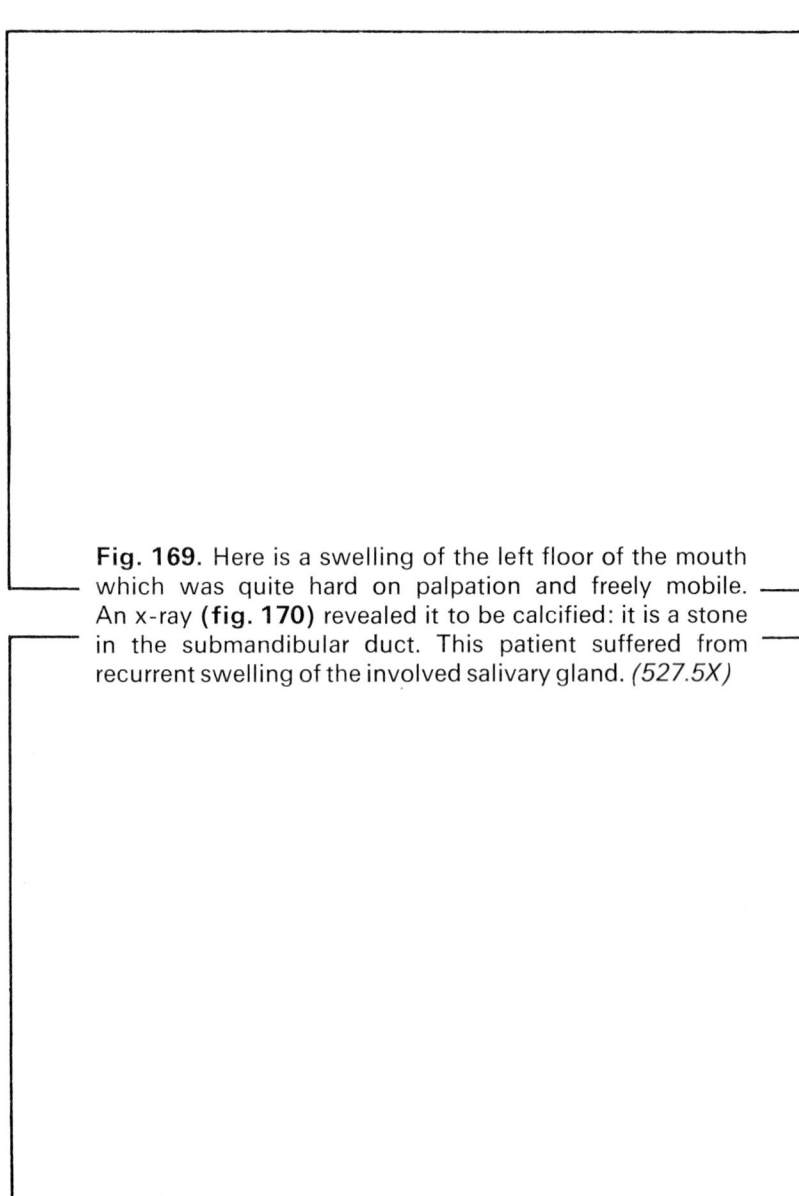

Fig. 169. Here is a swelling of the left floor of the mouth which was quite hard on palpation and freely mobile. An x-ray **(fig. 170)** revealed it to be calcified: it is a stone in the submandibular duct. This patient suffered from recurrent swelling of the involved salivary gland. *(527.5X)*

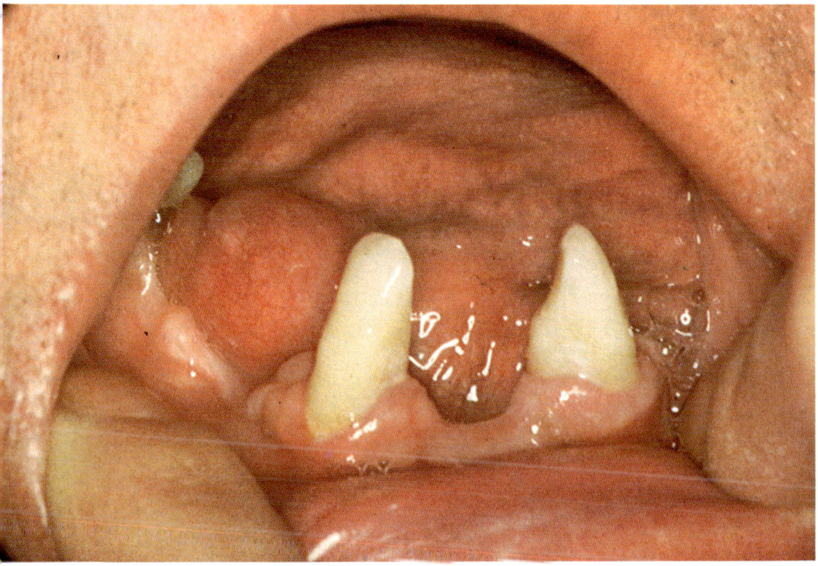

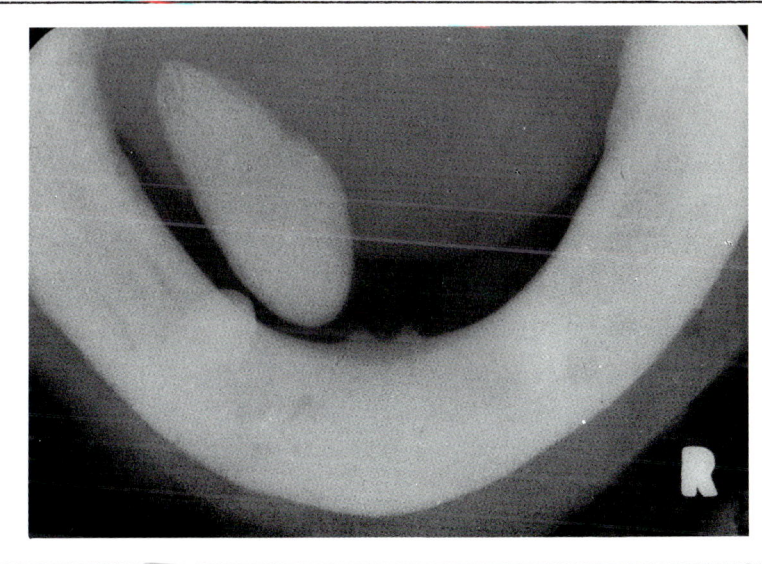

Fig. 171. Torus mandibularis — a horizontally disposed boss of bone on the lingual side of the mandible in the premolar region. Usually the exostosis is bilaterally symmetrical. *(526.91)*

Fig. 172. This x-ray shows a stone posteriorly in the submandibular duct behind and below the mylohyoid muscle. *(527.5X)*

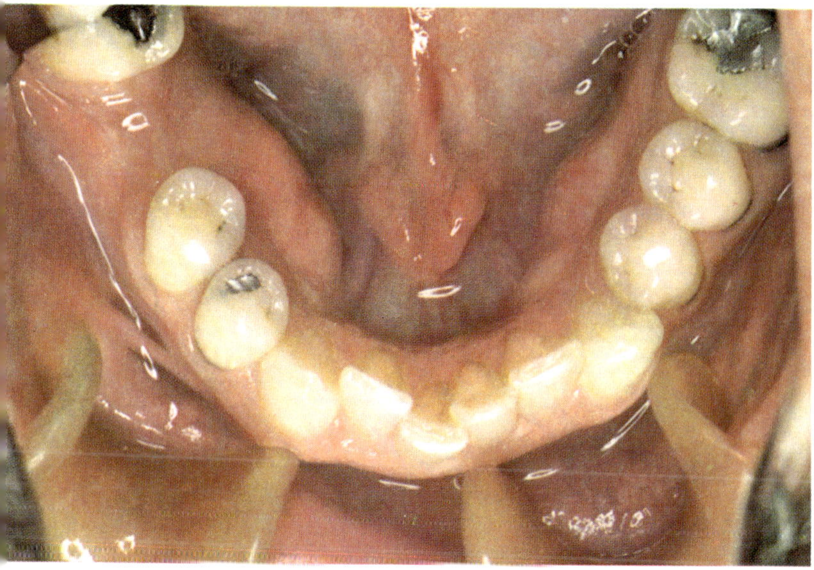

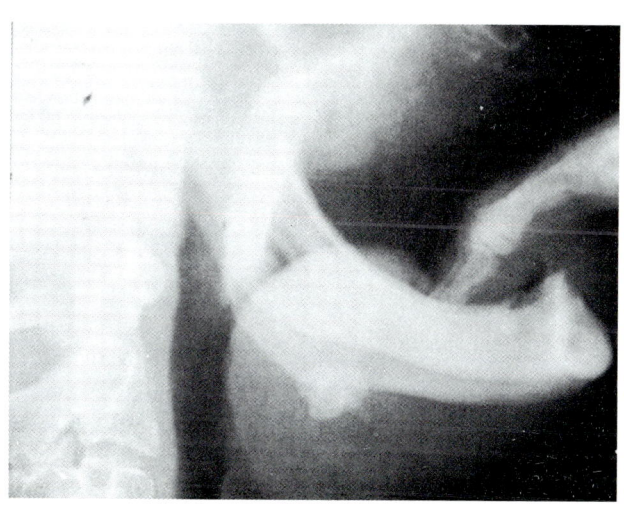

SECTION SIX: **PROSTHETIC PROBLEMS**

Fig. 173. A very extensive denture granuloma of the lower labial and left buccal sulcus. The "fit" of the flange between the outer two leaves of the hyperplastic tissue is well seen. *(528.90)*

Fig. 174. Epithelial inlay of the lower labial sulcus—the transplanted skin retains a more opaque appearance than oral mucosa.

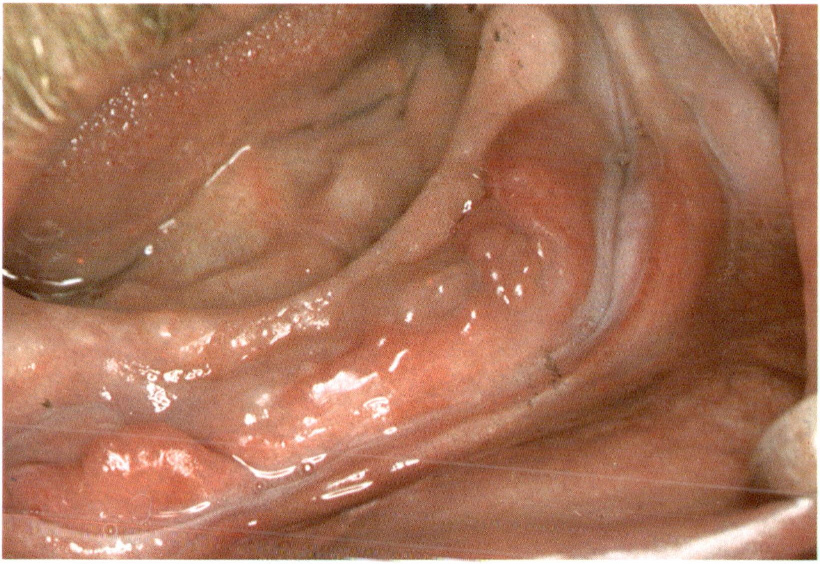

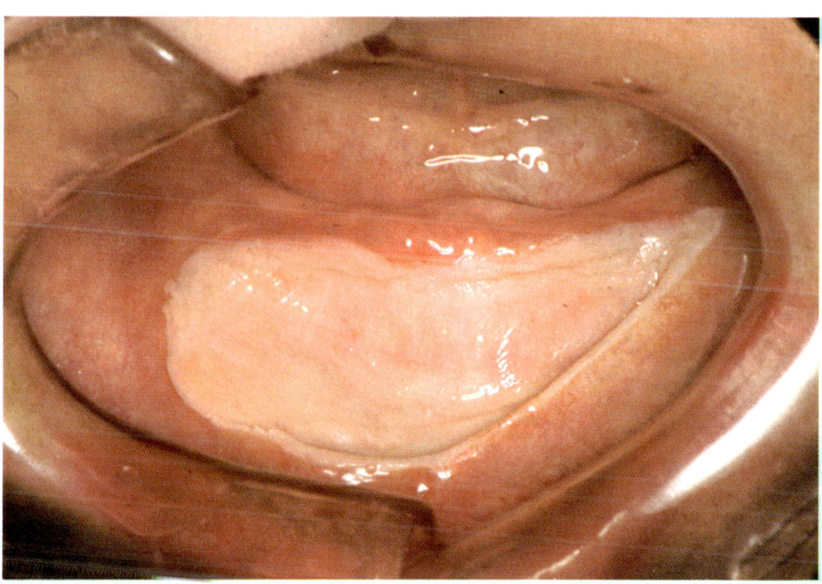

167

Fig. 175. A well-marked upper labial fraenum. *(750.87)*

Fig. 176. Buccal fraenum in the lower left premolar region in an edentulous patient. Such a high fraenal attachment causes a prosthetic problem and surgical excision of the band is indicated in order to provide a satisfactory base for a denture. *(750.87)*

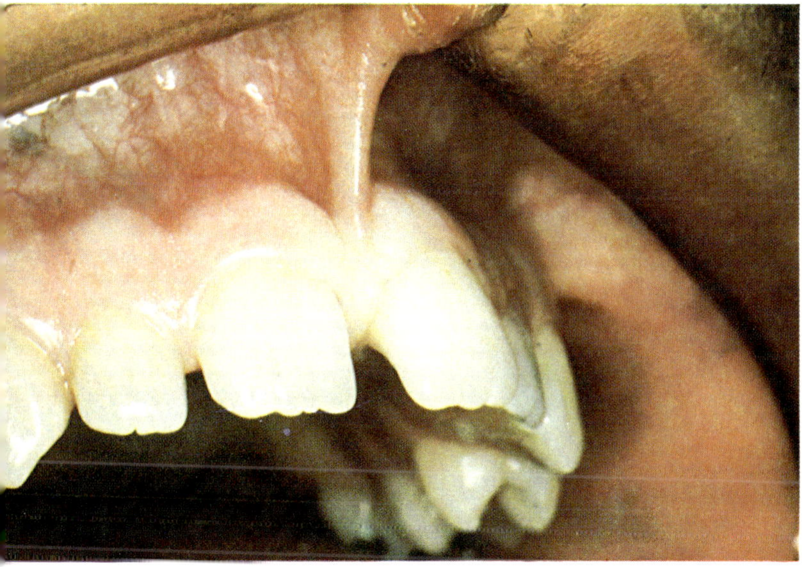

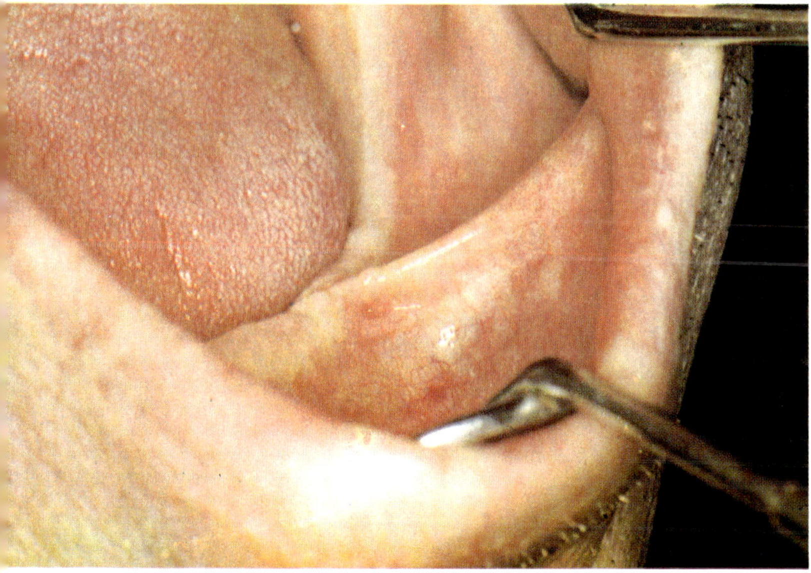

169

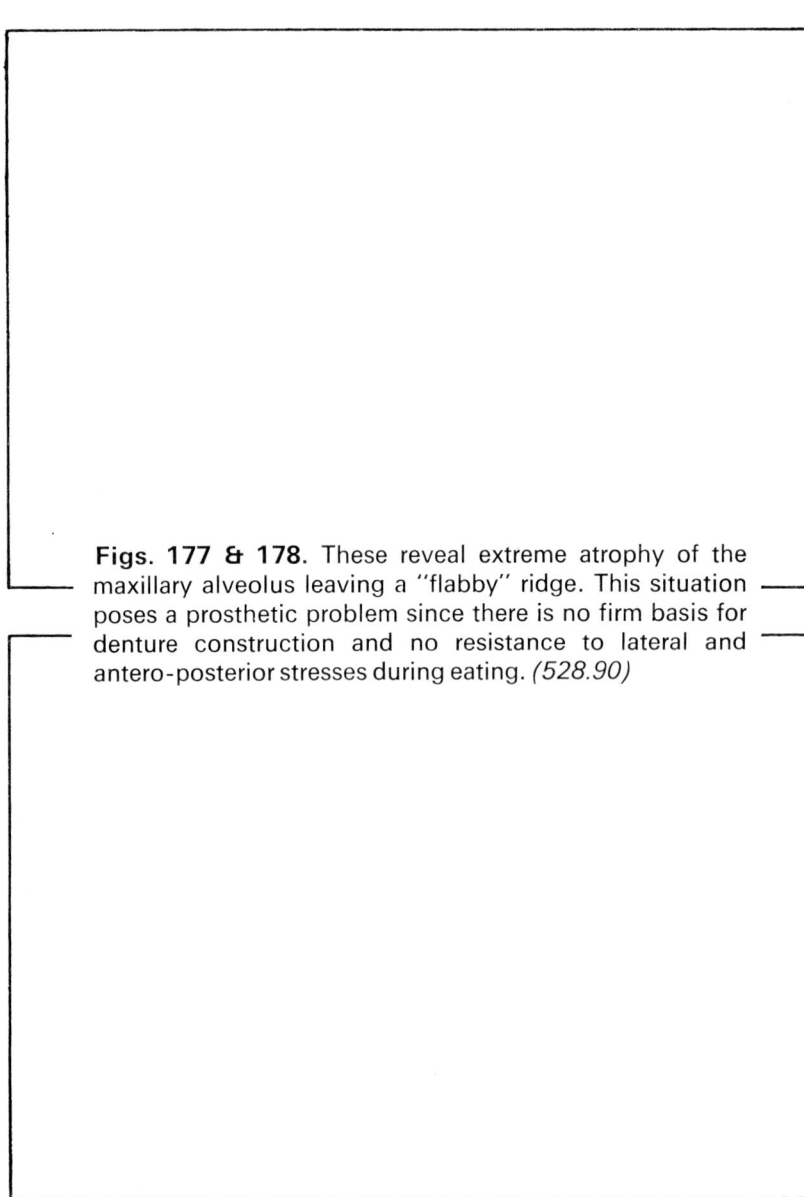

Figs. 177 & 178. These reveal extreme atrophy of the maxillary alveolus leaving a "flabby" ridge. This situation poses a prosthetic problem since there is no firm basis for denture construction and no resistance to lateral and antero-posterior stresses during eating. *(528.90)*

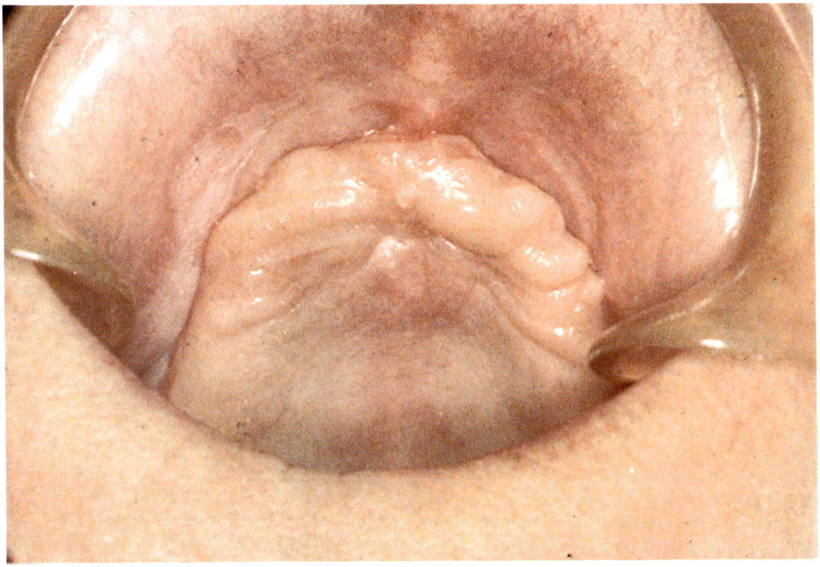

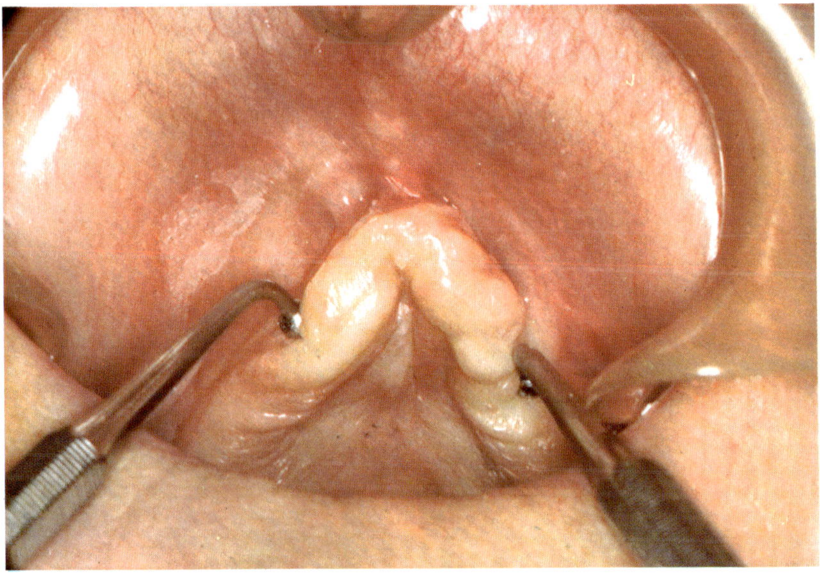

171

SECTION SEVEN: **THE PALATE**

Fig. 179. Torus palatinus. This is a very well-developed lobulated torus. A single smooth eminence is more usual. The mucosa over a torus is extremely thin and delicate. It is impossible to construct a satisfactory denture over such a lump. *(526.92)*

Fig. 180. Pleomorphic adenoma of the centre of the hard/soft palate junction. This lesion is firm to the touch but never bony hard like a torus. *(210.23)*

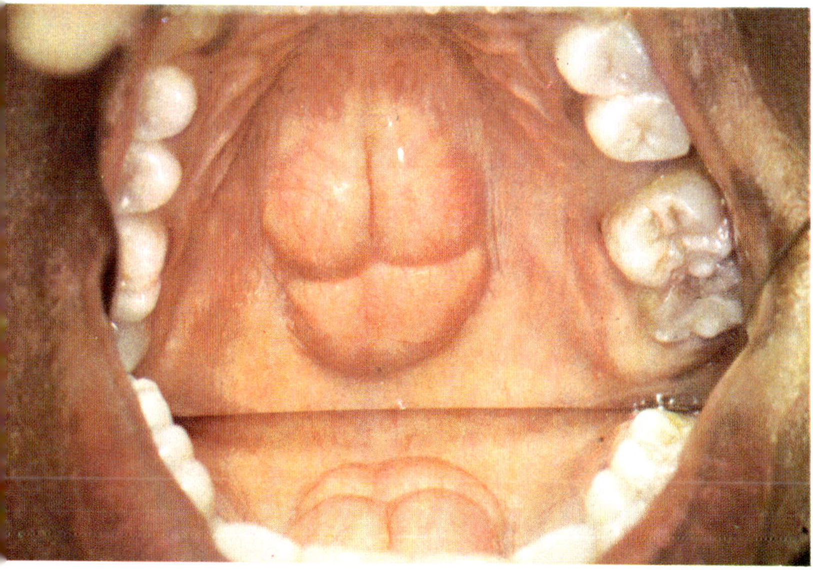

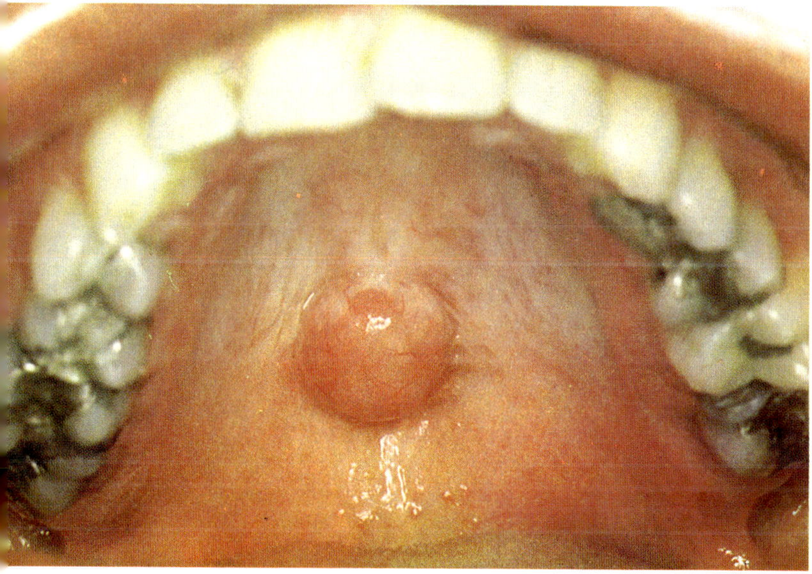

Fig. 181. This bluish spot in the centre of the palate was soft on palpation and was caused by a large median palatine cyst.

Fig. 182. The radiograph of the cyst. All the teeth were vital. *(526.11)*

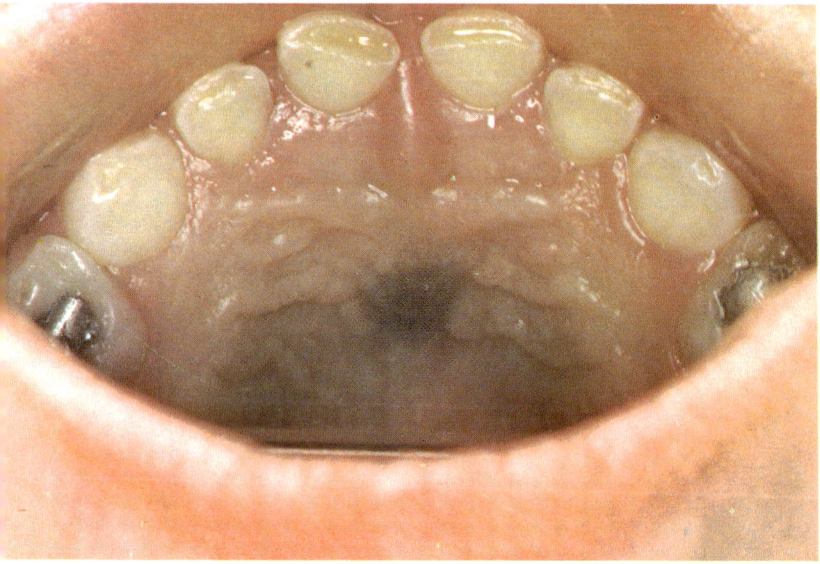

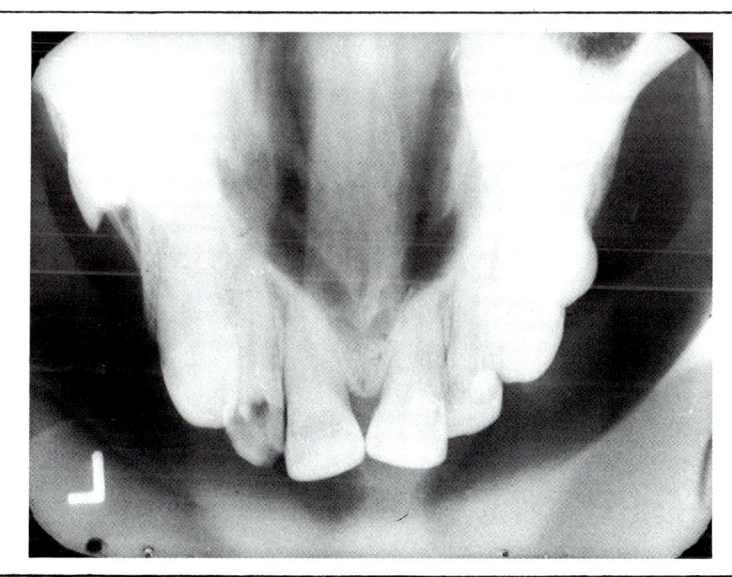

Fig. 183. Multiple small nodules in the vault of the hard palate characteristic of a condition termed inflammatory papillary hyperplasia. The aetiology is not known, but it seems to develop only in highly arched palates and beneath a denture. This patient was wearing a denture plate which covered the whole of the palate although replacing only four incisor teeth. *(528.90)*

Fig. 184. Cleft of the secondary palate here involving only the soft palate. *(749.01)*

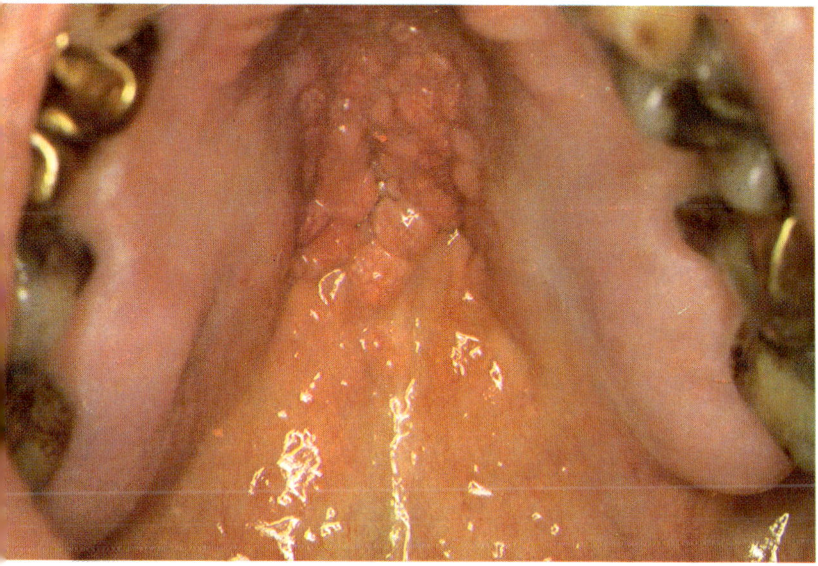

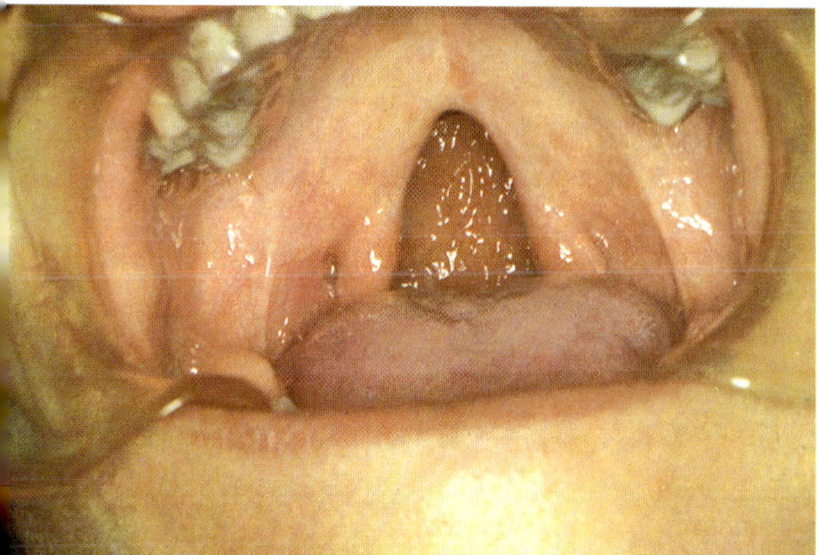

177

Fig. 185. This swelling of the palate is an abscess derived from periapical infection around a left maxillary lateral incisor. Pus usually localises near to the culpable tooth, but a palatal abscess on an upper lateral may occasionally point some distance away from the focus, namely, at the junction of hard and soft palates. Palatal abscesses are usually very painful. *(522.5X)*

Fig. 186. "Leaf" fibro-epithelial polyp of the palate. The lesion arises from a very narrow pedicle and is pressed flat by the upper denture, only hanging down on removal of the prosthesis. *(528.90)*

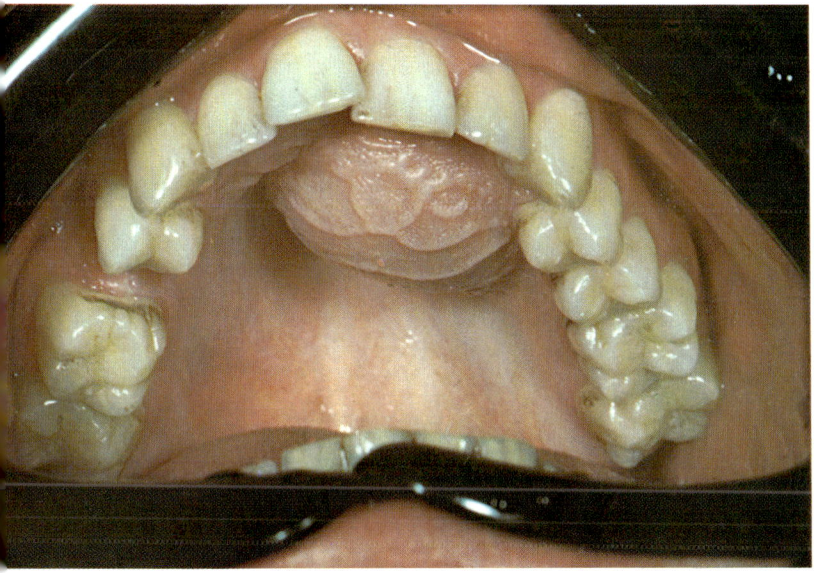

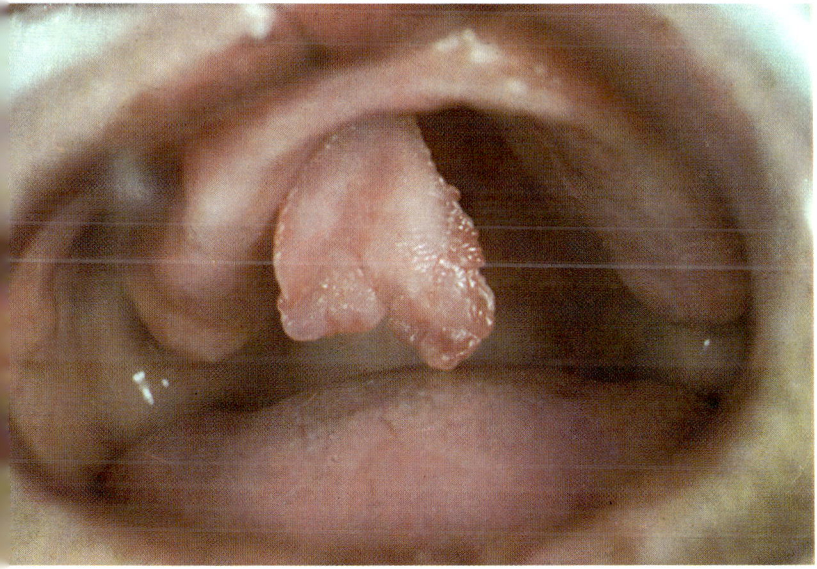

179

Fig. 187. An ulcer of the posterior part of the hard palate thought to be traumatic. In this site particularly an ulceration not infrequently develops for which a cause cannot be established. This ulcer healed without treatment, but it is important with atypical ulcers to exclude syphilis as a cause.

Fig. 188. A similar lesion. *(N873.7)*

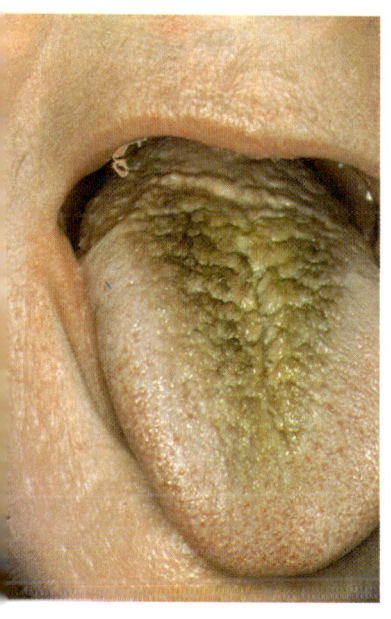
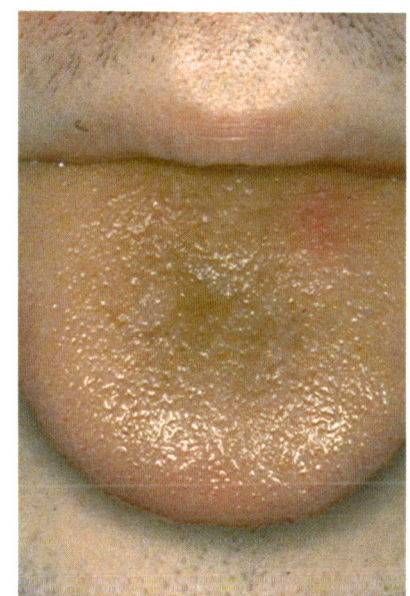
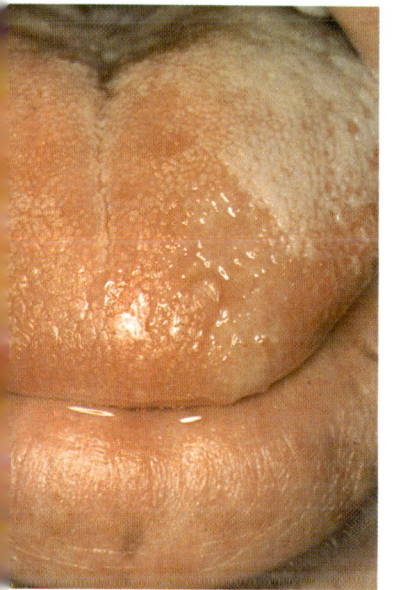
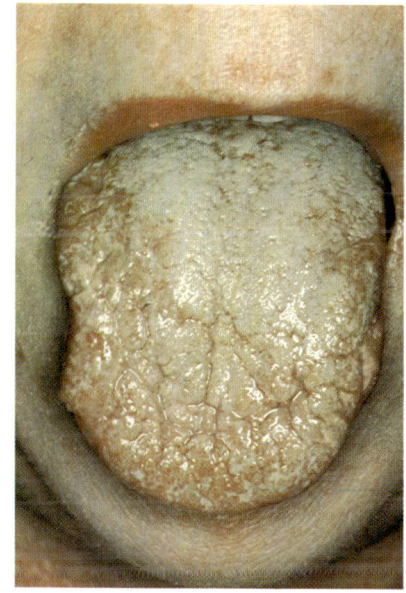

191

Fig. 205. The same case as the one preceding. The small ulcer is a squamous cell carcinoma. *(095.X2; 141.2X)*

Fig. 206. Partial atrophy of the left side of the tongue due to a lesion of the hypoglossal nerve. *(355.X1)*

Fig. 207. An atrophic pale tongue typical of iron deficiency anaemia. *(280.X0)*

Fig. 208. A rapidly growing lesion of the left side of the tongue which proved to be a sarcoma. Sarcoma of the mouth is extremely uncommon compared with squamous-cell carcinoma. *(171.0X)*

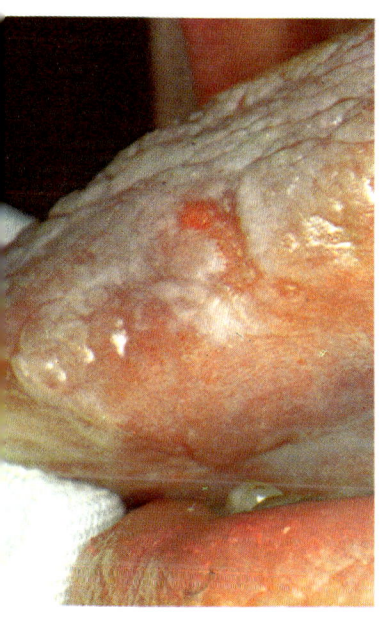
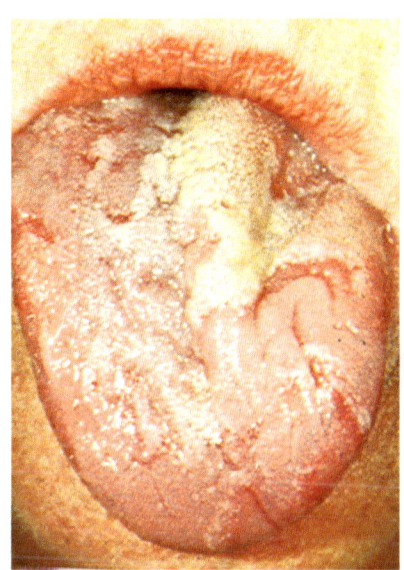
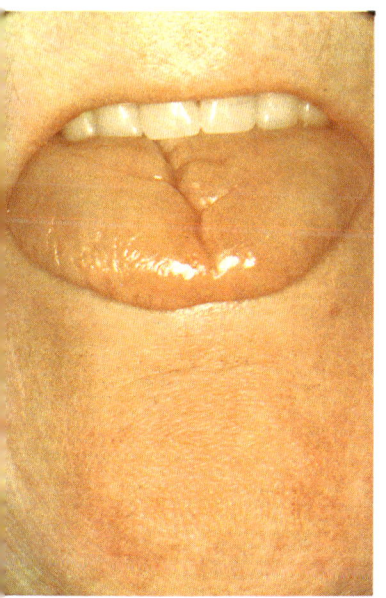
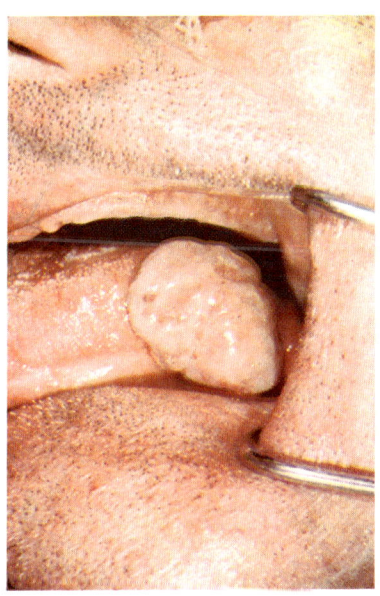

Fig. 209. This dry wrinkled and discoloured tongue is secondary to the xerostomia of the sicca syndrome. *(734.90)*

Fig. 210. The same patient with atrophic mucosa and extensive cervical caries. *(734.90)*

Fig. 211. A haemangioma of the left side of the tongue. *(227.X0)*

Fig. 212. Multiple neurofibromatous nodules in von Recklinghausen's neurofibromatosis. *(743.40)*

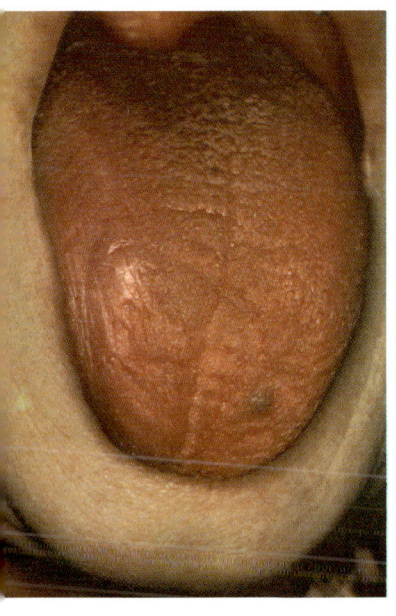
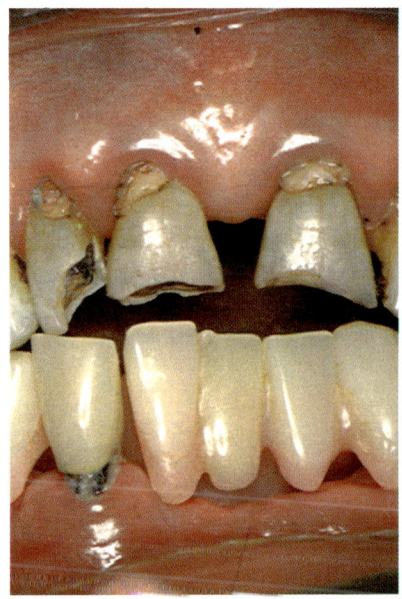
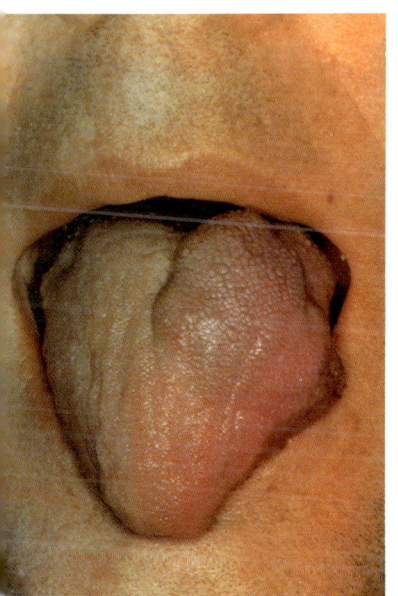
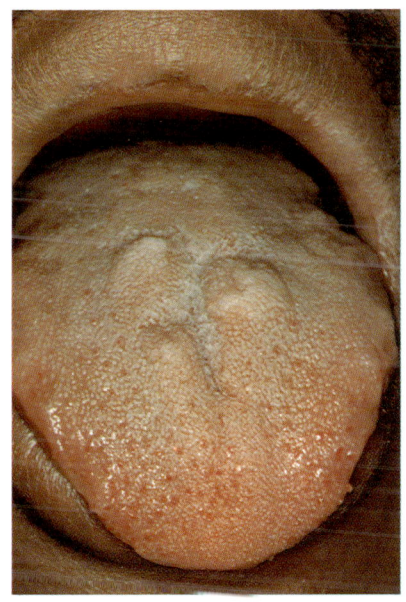

195

SECTION NINE: **RADIOPACITIES and RADIOLUCENCIES**

Figs. 213 & 214. These x-rays show an osteoma of the mandible attached to the lower border. *(213.XO)*

Figs. 215 & 216. This x-ray shows what appear to be multiple radiopacities in the mandible. The lateral oblique view **(fig. 216),** however, indicates that they lie outside the mandible. They are, in fact, calcified lymph nodes due to healed tuberculous lymphadenitis. *(017.10)*

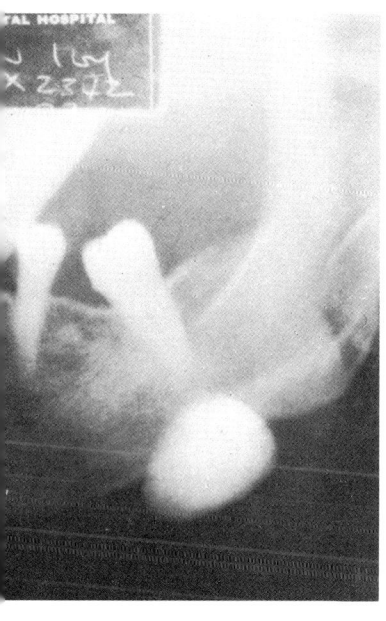
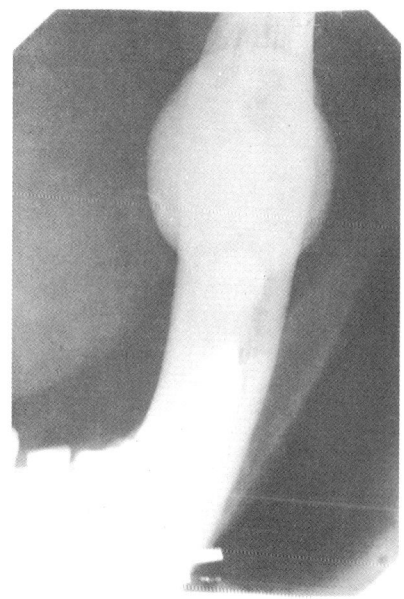
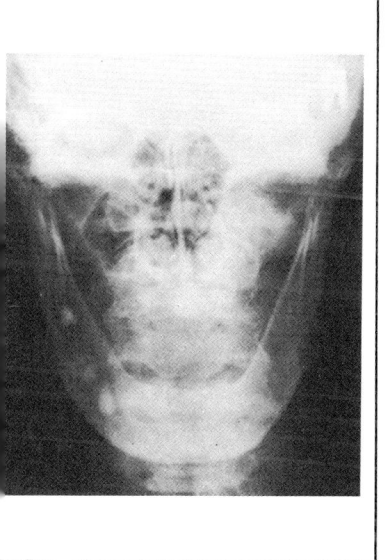
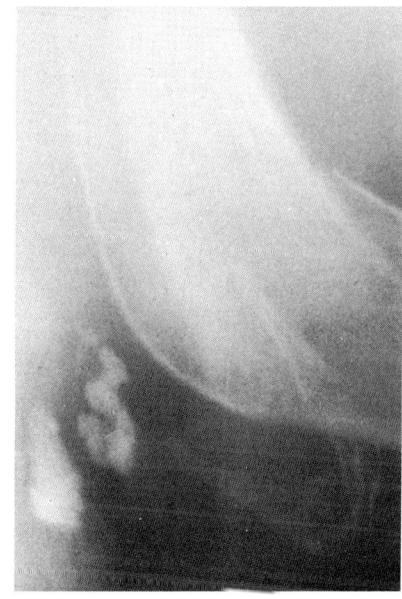

197

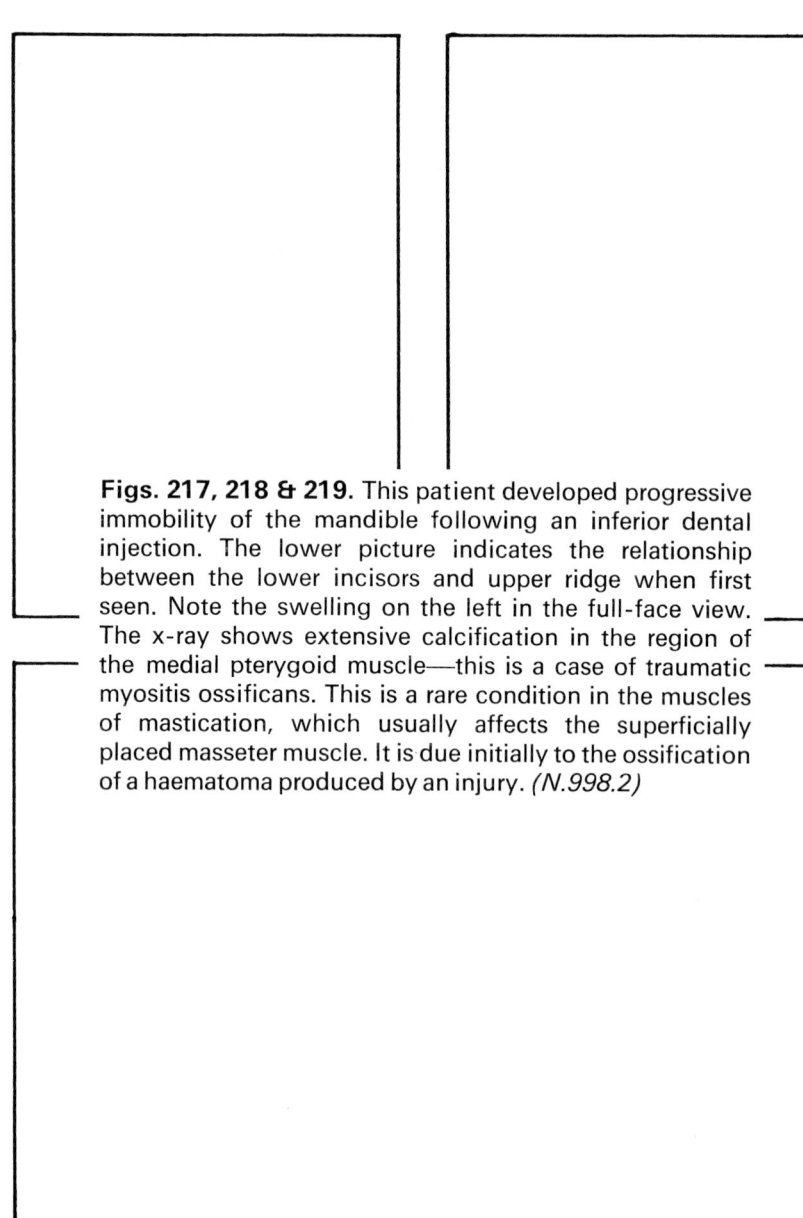

Figs. 217, 218 & 219. This patient developed progressive immobility of the mandible following an inferior dental injection. The lower picture indicates the relationship between the lower incisors and upper ridge when first seen. Note the swelling on the left in the full-face view. The x-ray shows extensive calcification in the region of the medial pterygoid muscle—this is a case of traumatic myositis ossificans. This is a rare condition in the muscles of mastication, which usually affects the superficially placed masseter muscle. It is due initially to the ossification of a haematoma produced by an injury. *(N.998.2)*

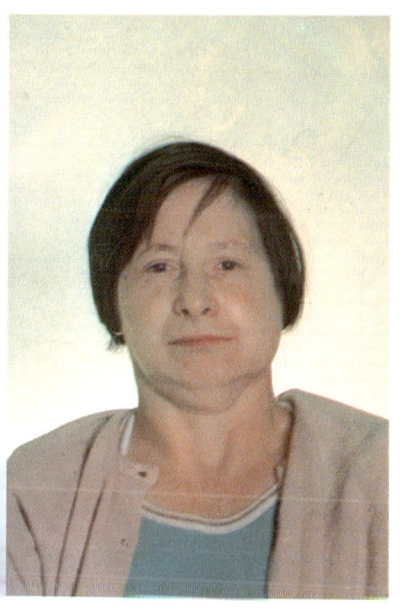
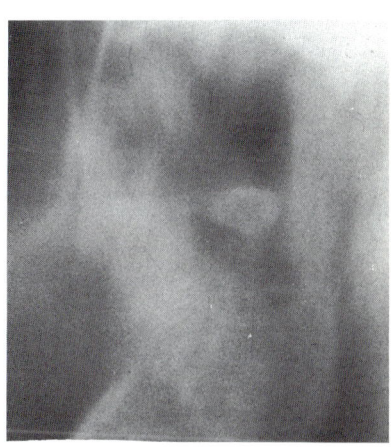

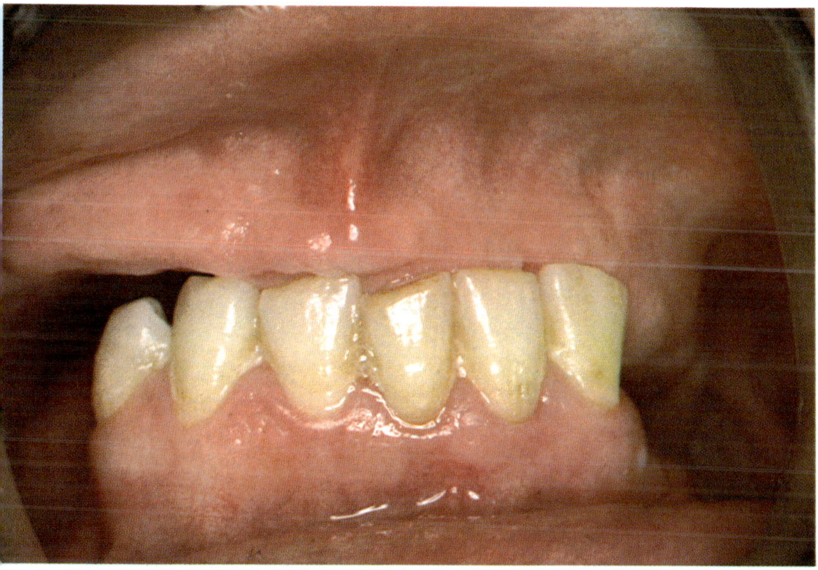

199

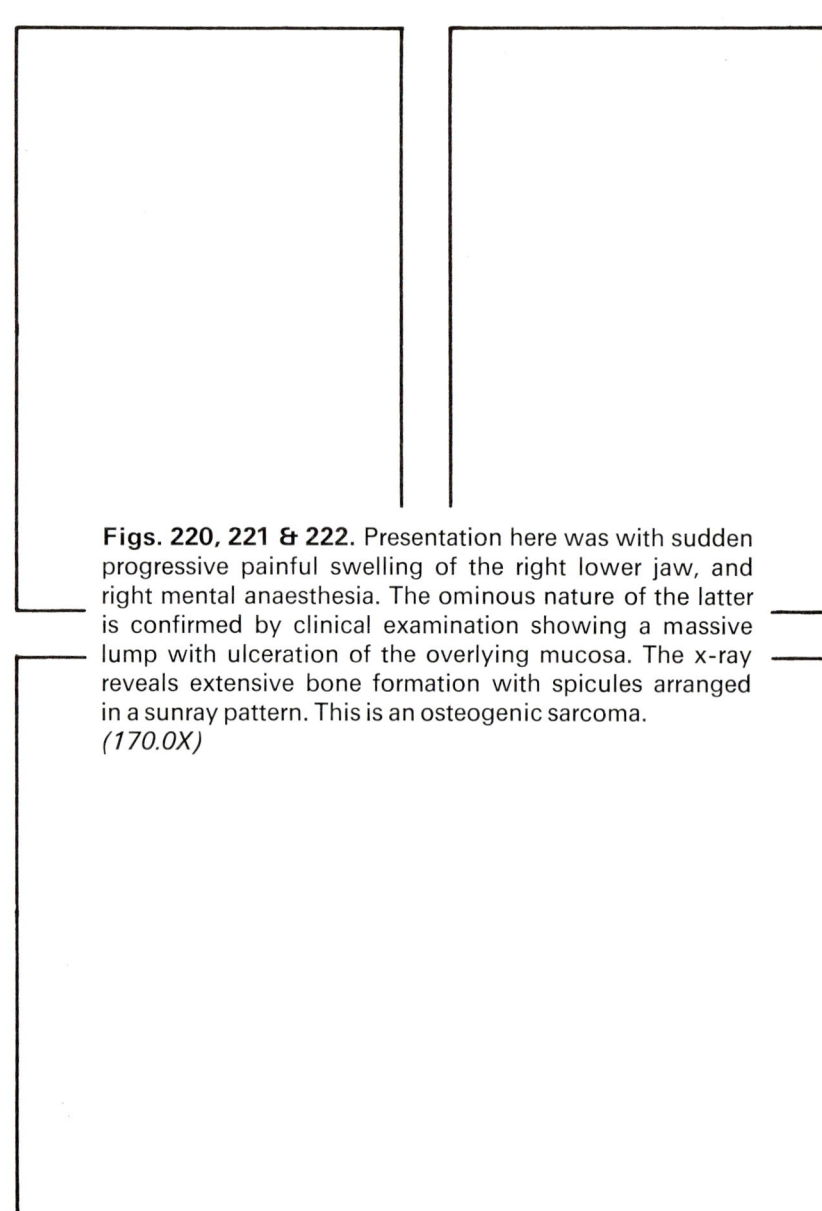

Figs. 220, 221 & 222. Presentation here was with sudden progressive painful swelling of the right lower jaw, and right mental anaesthesia. The ominous nature of the latter is confirmed by clinical examination showing a massive lump with ulceration of the overlying mucosa. The x-ray reveals extensive bone formation with spicules arranged in a sunray pattern. This is an osteogenic sarcoma.
(170.0X)

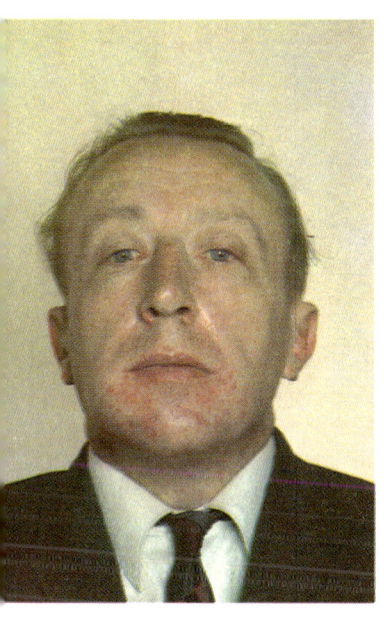
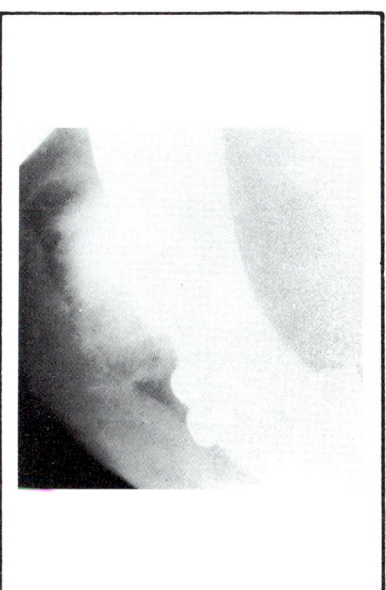

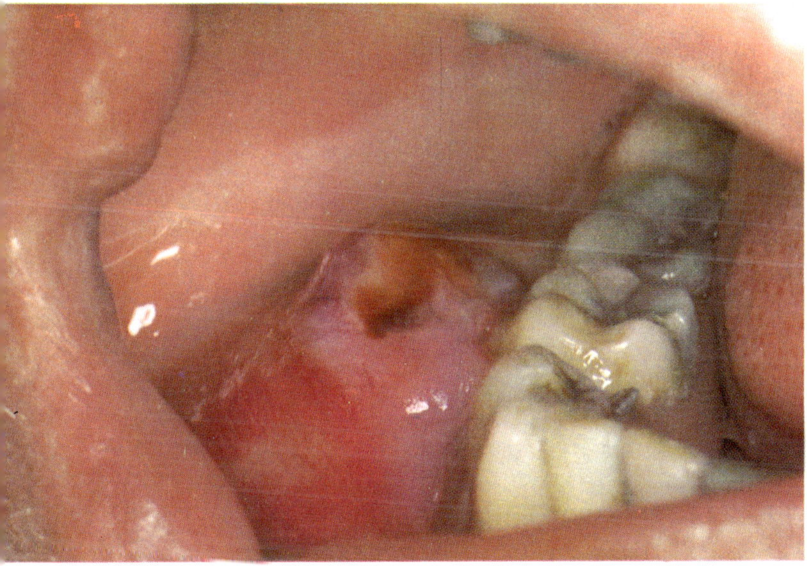

Fig. 223. The parent of this young patient noticed a swelling in his mouth. Examination revealed expansion of the mandible and a bluish cystic swelling is visible. X-ray confirmed a dentigerous cyst of the right first premolar. *(526.02)*

Fig. 224. This soft cystic swelling in the floor of the mouth is a ranula—the name given to a large mucous extravasation cyst derived from the sublingual salivary gland. *(527.61)*

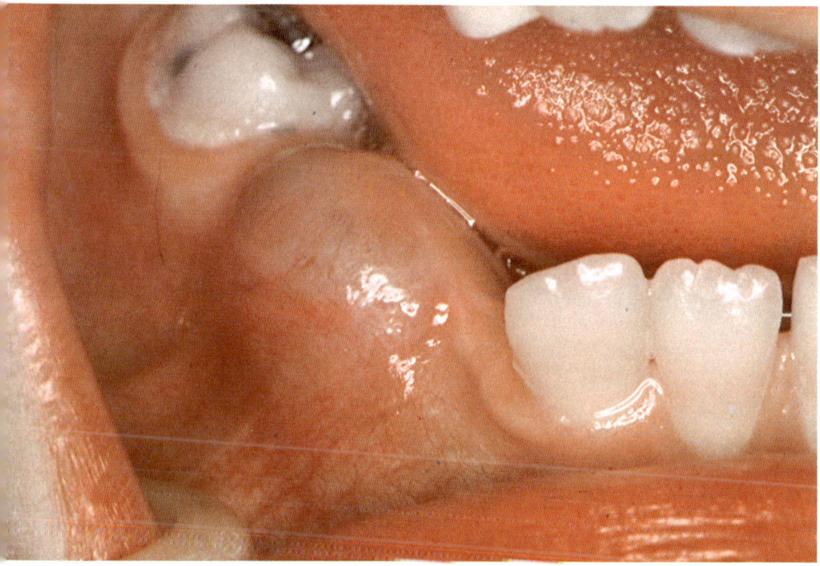

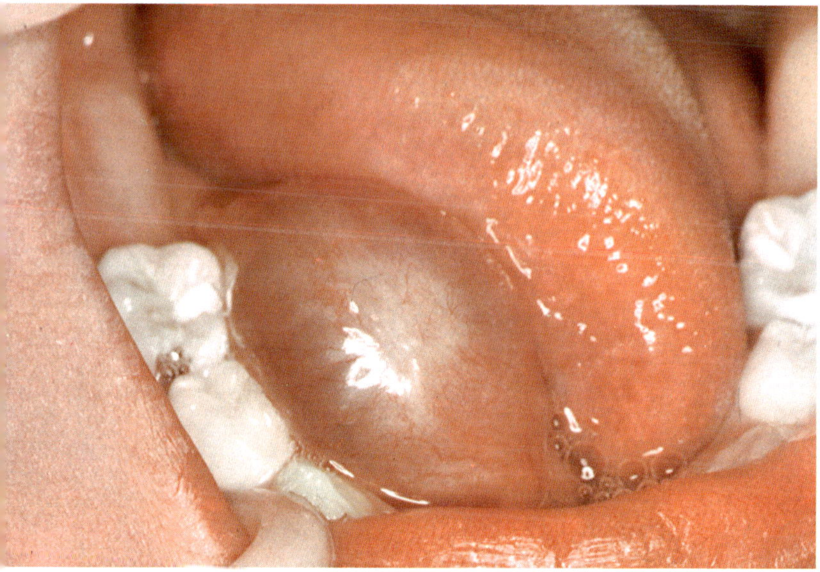

203

Fig. 225. A lateral oblique x-ray of the mandible shows the typical feature of a residual cyst of the mandible. Note the smooth outline of the radiolucency with its margin of increased radiopacity; the latter is often referred to as the cortical line. *(522.82)*

Fig. 226. Another radiolucency of the mandible with a slightly scalloped margin and no increase in bone density at the periphery. The tooth roots are not displaced and all teeth are vital. This is simply a hole in the bone glorified by its title of haemorrhagic (solitary, traumatic) bone cyst. It is almost as if part of the cortico-cancellous structure of the mandible had been hollowed out, leaving the teeth and their lamina dura unaffected. The neurovascular bundle courses through the cavity bereft of its bony sheath. *(526.21)*

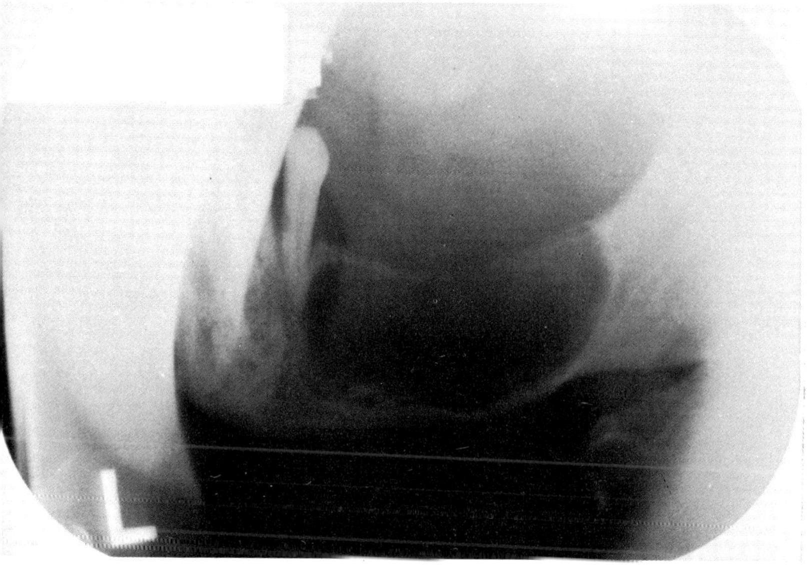

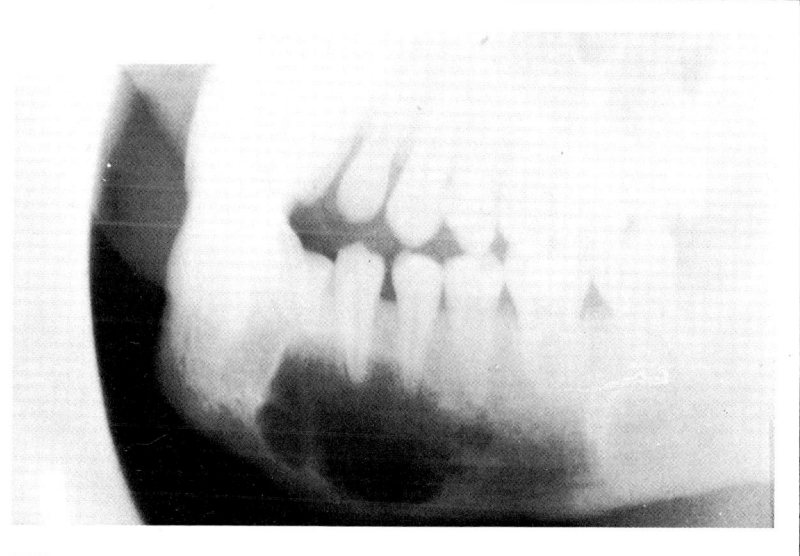

Fig. 227. A further example of a residual cyst of the mandible showing typical clinical features. *(522.82)*

Fig. 228. The classical radiographic appearance of odontogenic cysts—namely, an ovoid radiolucency with a narrow radiopaque periphery—is well demonstrated in this view. *(522.82)*

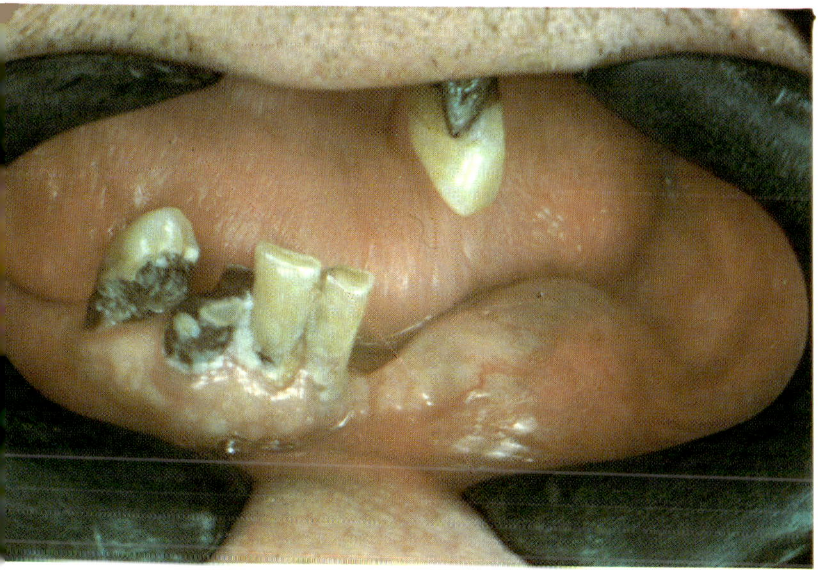

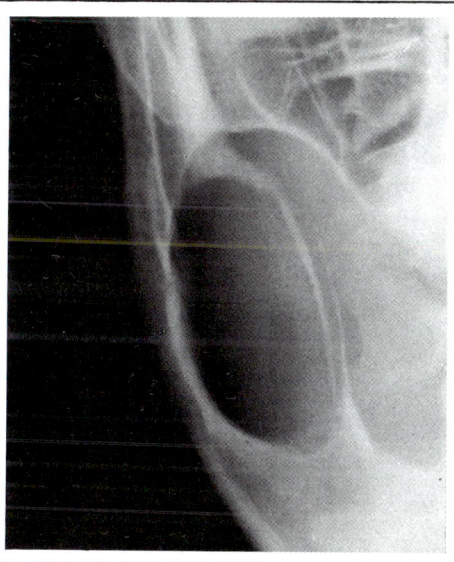

Fig. 229. Another x-ray of a dental cyst—but this time the lesion is extremely large. It has destroyed much of the ascending ramus, the anterior border of which has ballooned forwards. *(526.01)*

Fig. 230. Here is depicted an odontogenic cyst which is deeply lobulated with septae of bone partly separating its compartments. Although the cyst is extensive, it is largely confined within the original shape of the mandible. This is a typical odontogenic keratocyst, although ameloblastoma must be excluded. *(526.01)*

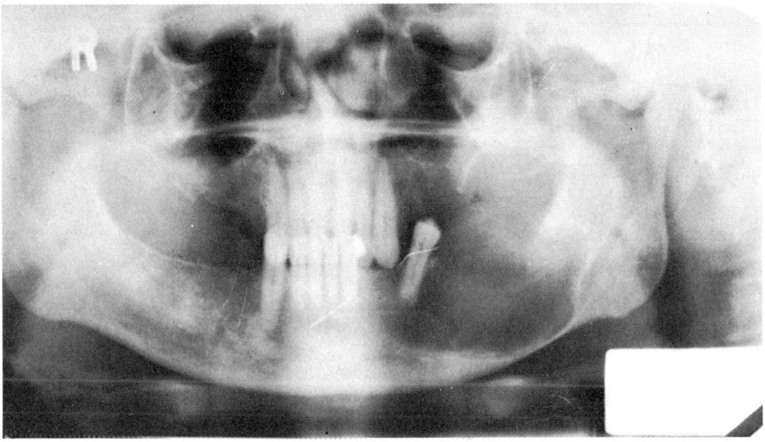

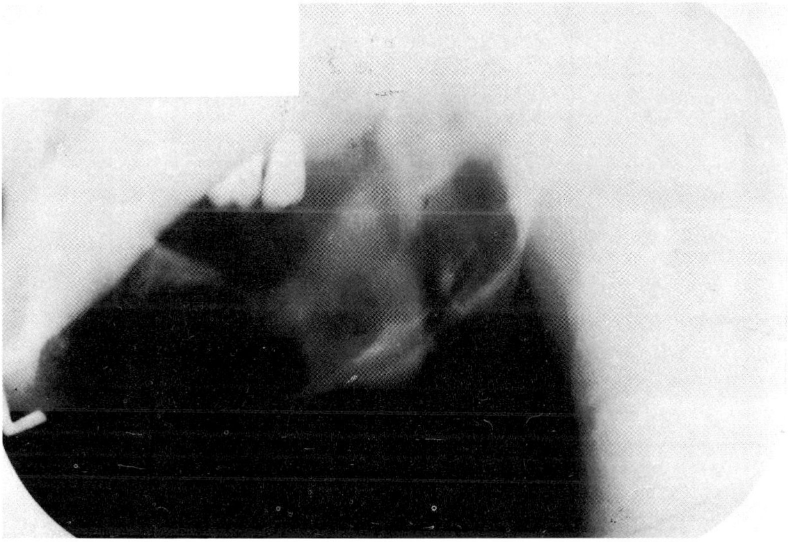

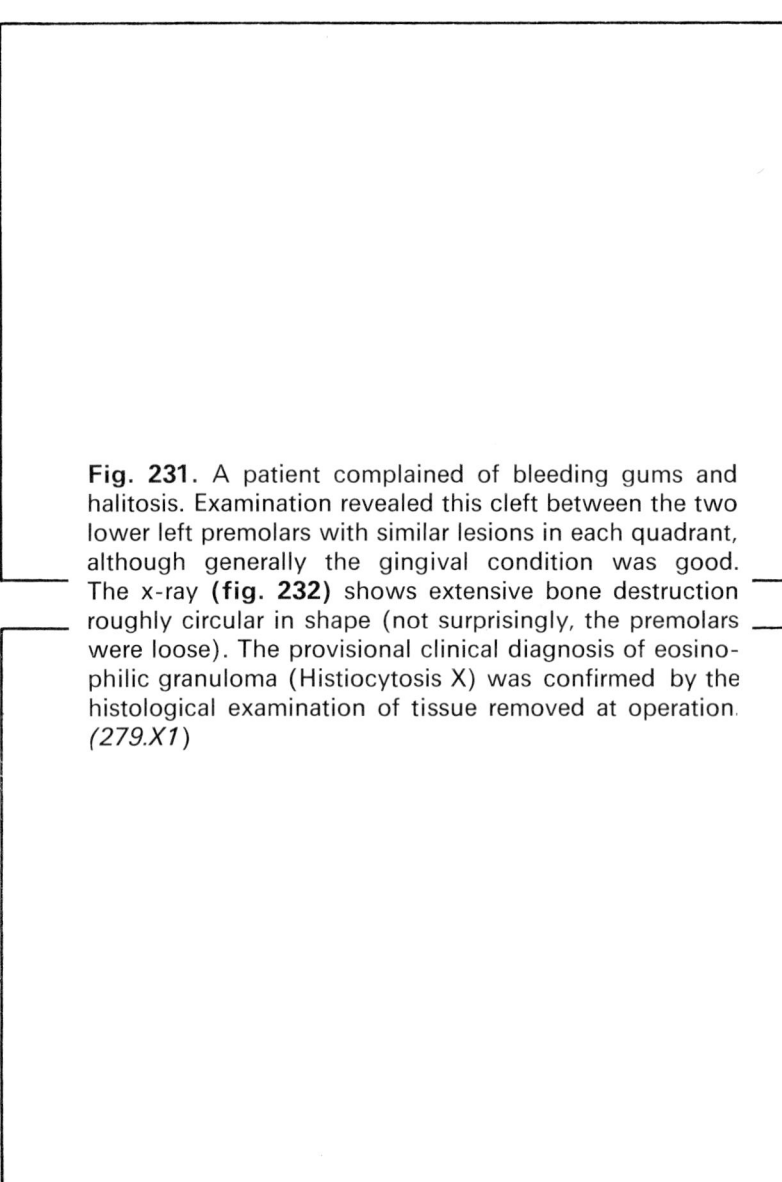

Fig. 231. A patient complained of bleeding gums and halitosis. Examination revealed this cleft between the two lower left premolars with similar lesions in each quadrant, although generally the gingival condition was good. The x-ray **(fig. 232)** shows extensive bone destruction roughly circular in shape (not surprisingly, the premolars were loose). The provisional clinical diagnosis of eosinophilic granuloma (Histiocytosis X) was confirmed by the histological examination of tissue removed at operation. *(279.X1)*

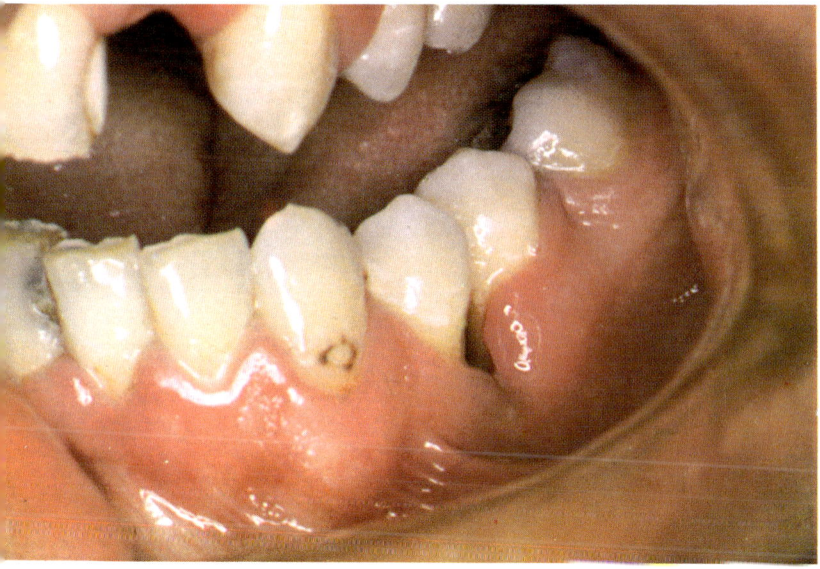

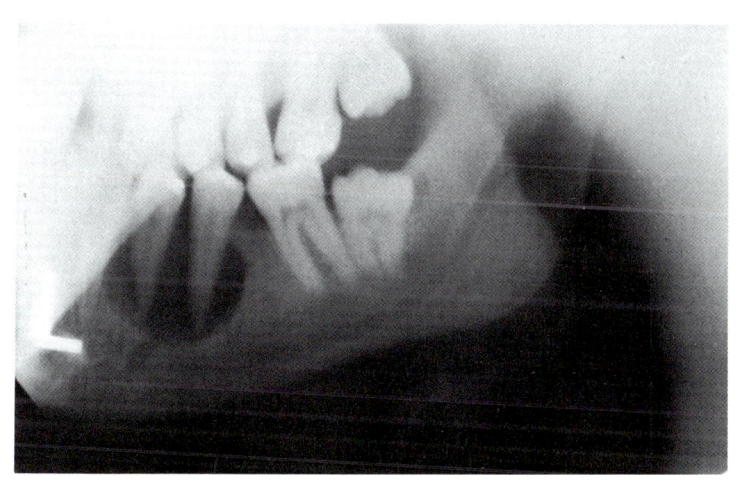

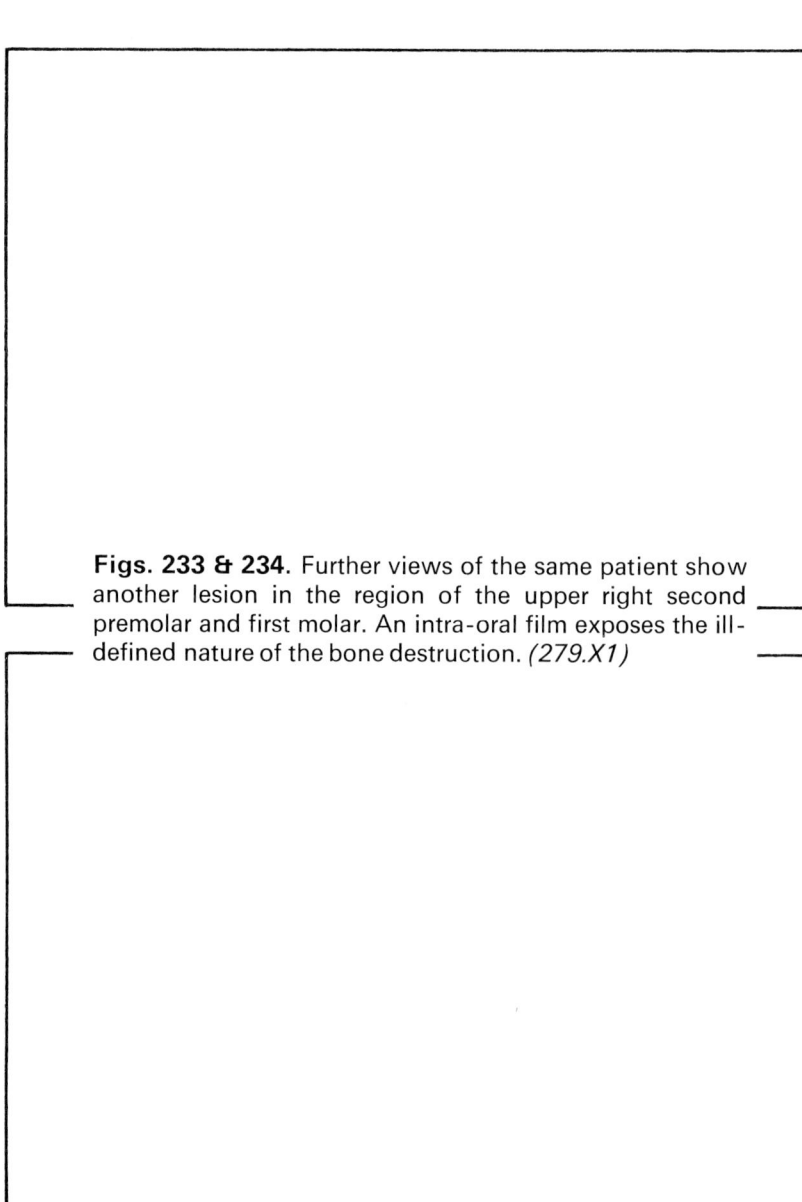

Figs. 233 & 234. Further views of the same patient show another lesion in the region of the upper right second premolar and first molar. An intra-oral film exposes the ill-defined nature of the bone destruction. *(279.X1)*

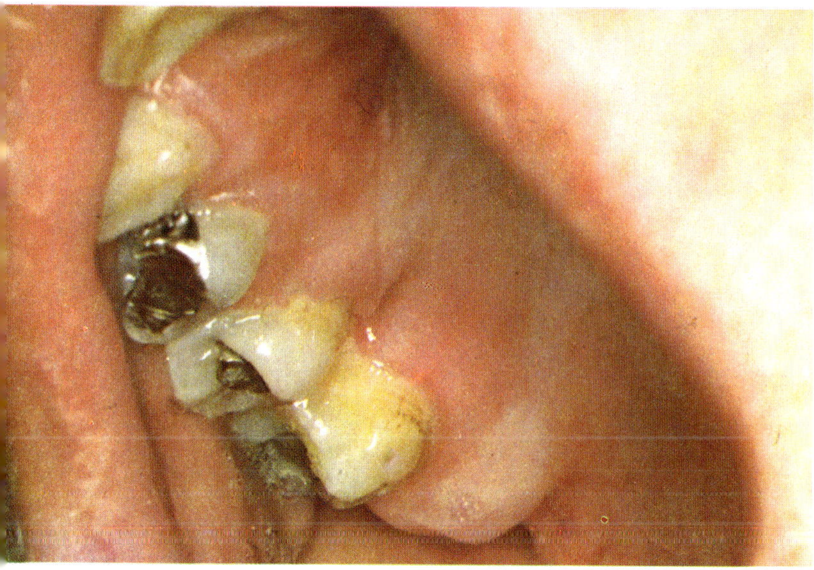

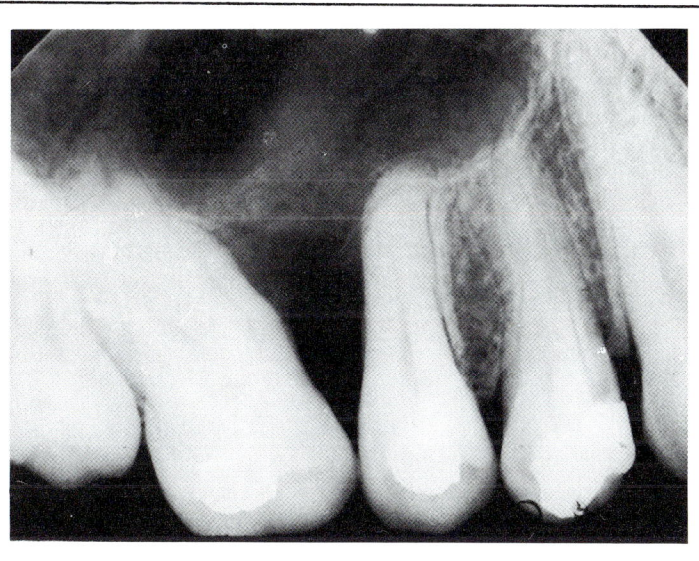

Fig. 235. An x-ray showing extensive expansion of the mandible both buccally and lingually. This is a myxofibroma. It could also be a giant-cell granuloma or fibrous dysplasia of bone. The only means of distinguishing between them is by biopsy. *(213.X0)*

Fig. 236. This diffuse osteolytic lesion of the mandible is due to Histiocytosis X. *(279.X1)*

Fig. 237. An osteolytic area of the mandible with a poorly defined margin. Excision of the lesion revealed it to be a giant-cell granuloma, but the serum calcium was elevated. It should, therefore, be designated as a ''brown tumour'' of hyperparathyroid bone disease. *(252.V0)*

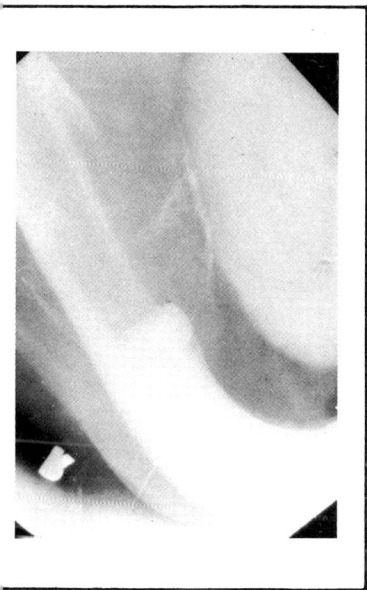
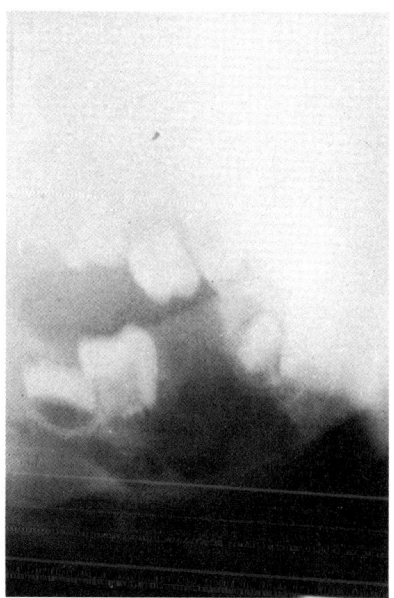
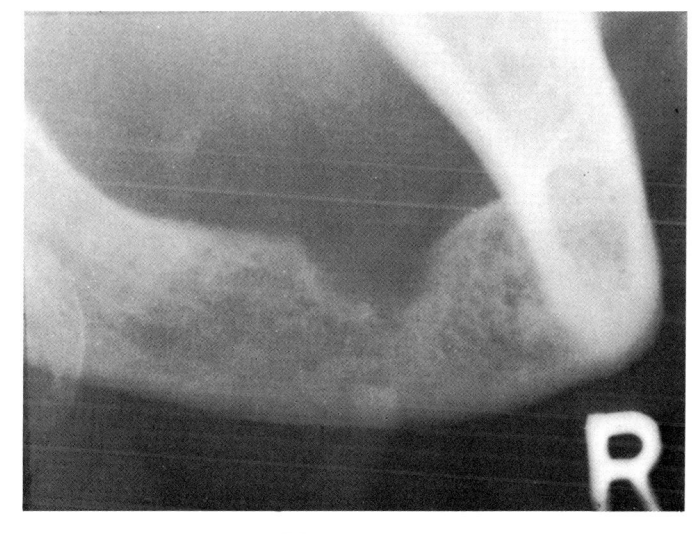

Fig. 238.

Fig. 239.

Figs. 238, 239 & 240. Fig. 238 is an intra-oral x-ray. **Fig. 240** below is the lateral oblique film of the same case, whose clinical picture is shown in **Fig. 165**. The resorption of the mandible is due to invasion by the squamous carcinoma. There is no periosteal new bone formation—the mandible looks "moth-eaten". For comparison, **Fig. 239** shows an extensive destructive lesion of the mandible of a child. This presented as a painful swelling for which the lower right second deciduous molar was removed, in the erroneous belief that it was abscessed. Persistence of the swelling led to biopsy which indicated a diagnosis of Histiocytosis X. Other lesions subsequently occurred in other parts of the skeleton. The x-ray shows bone solution, but a periosteal reaction is evident. *(279.X1)*

Fig. 240.

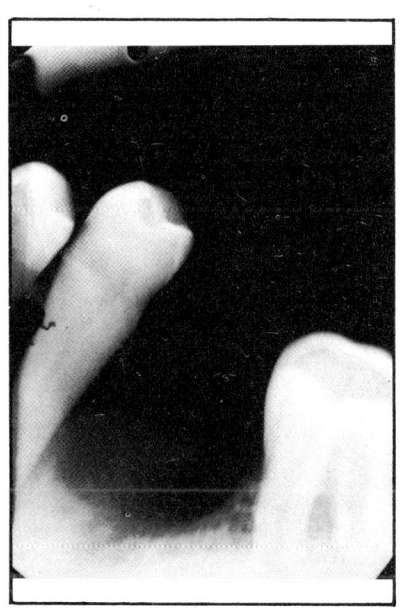
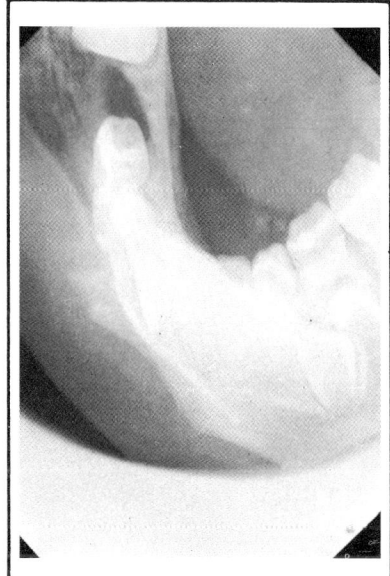

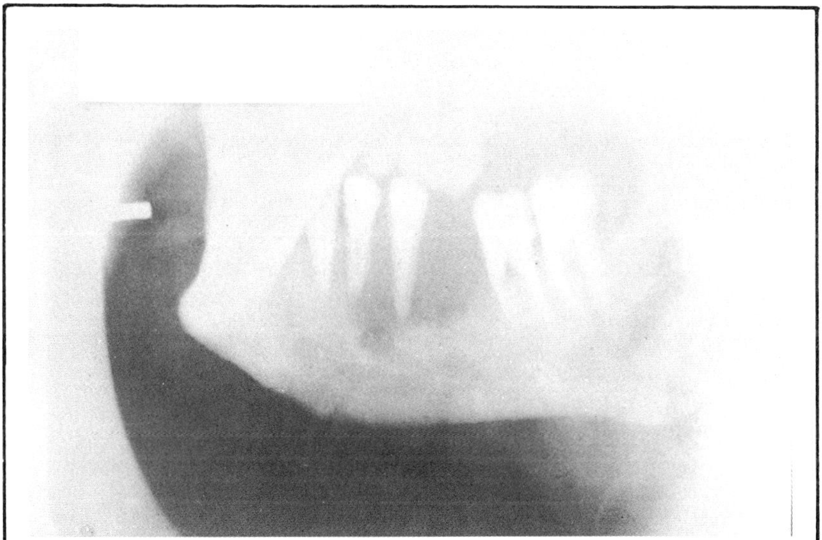

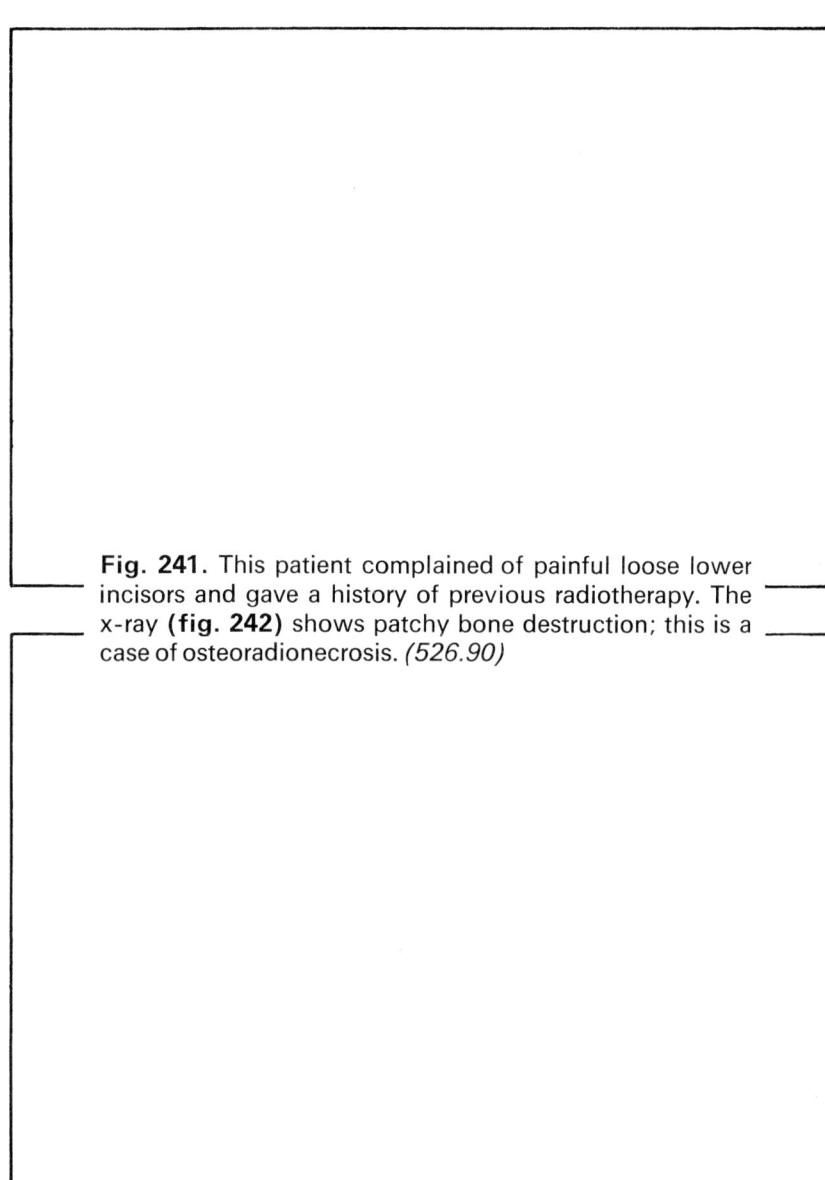

Fig. 241. This patient complained of painful loose lower incisors and gave a history of previous radiotherapy. The x-ray **(fig. 242)** shows patchy bone destruction; this is a case of osteoradionecrosis. *(526.90)*

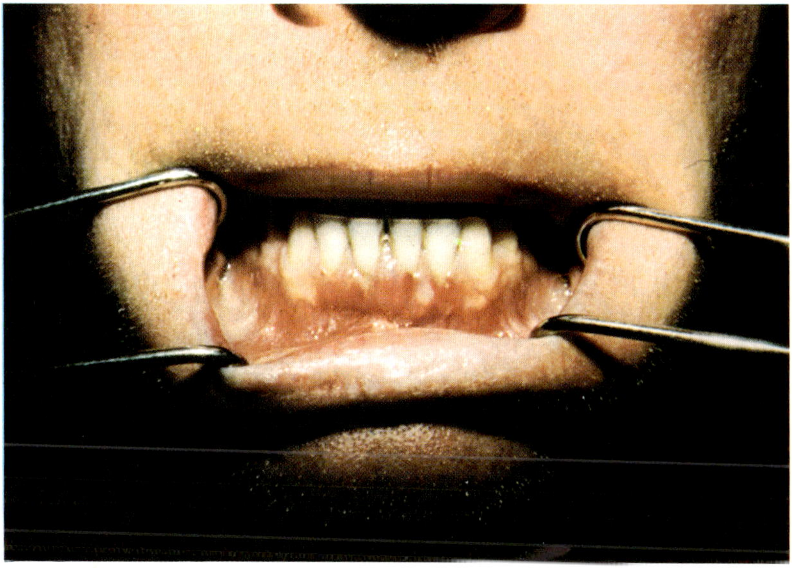

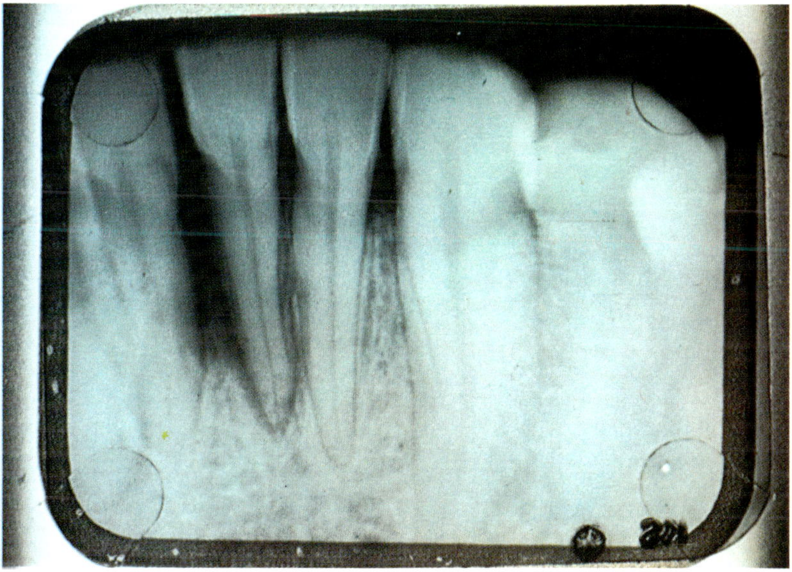

210

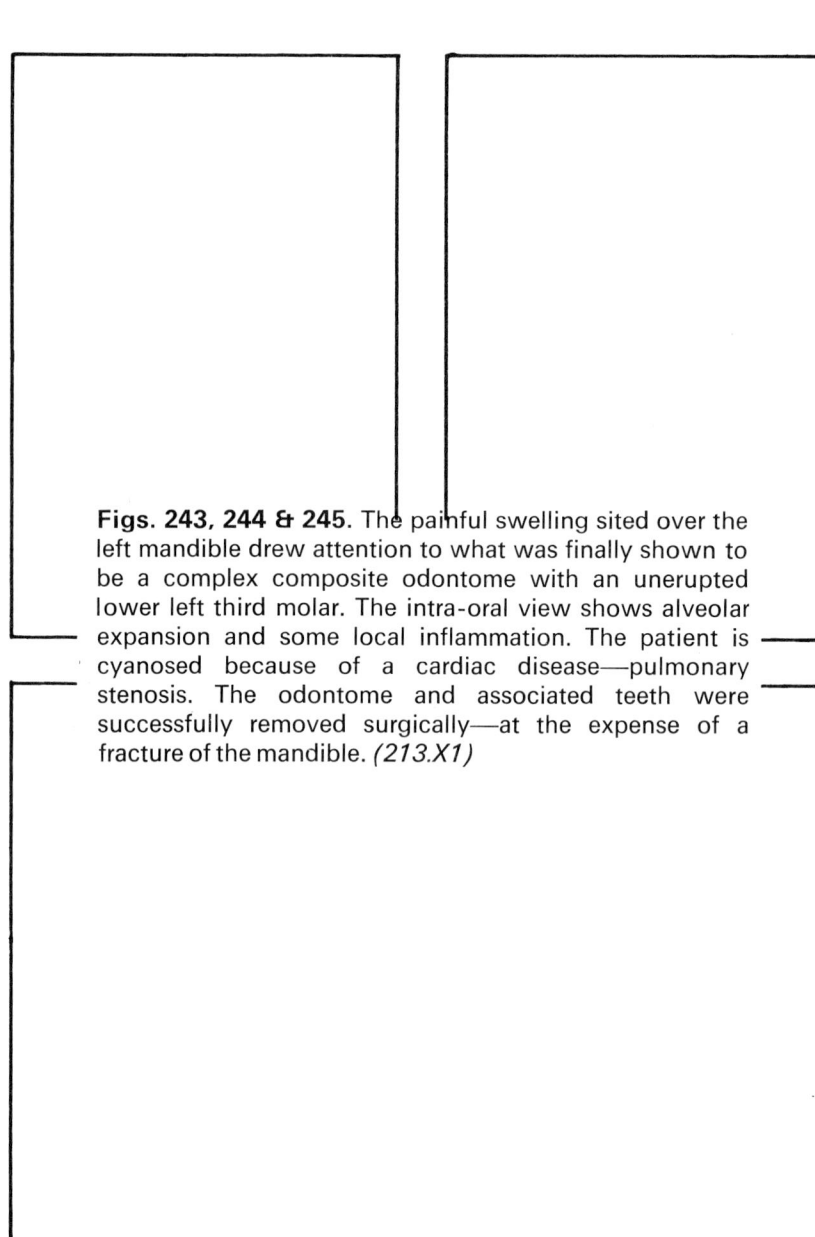

Figs. 243, 244 & 245. The painful swelling sited over the left mandible drew attention to what was finally shown to be a complex composite odontome with an unerupted lower left third molar. The intra-oral view shows alveolar expansion and some local inflammation. The patient is cyanosed because of a cardiac disease—pulmonary stenosis. The odontome and associated teeth were successfully removed surgically—at the expense of a fracture of the mandible. *(213.X1)*

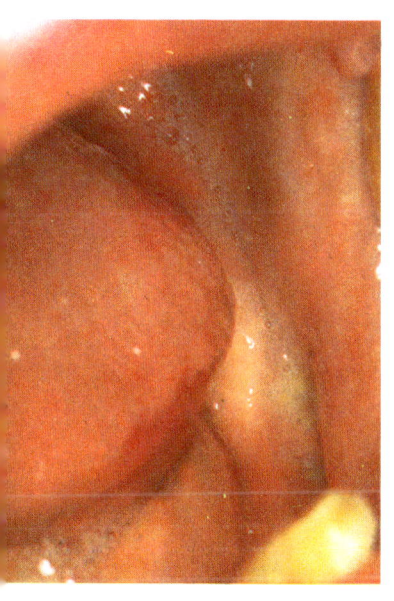
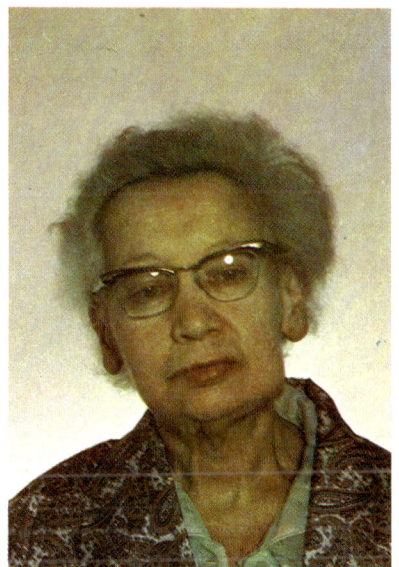

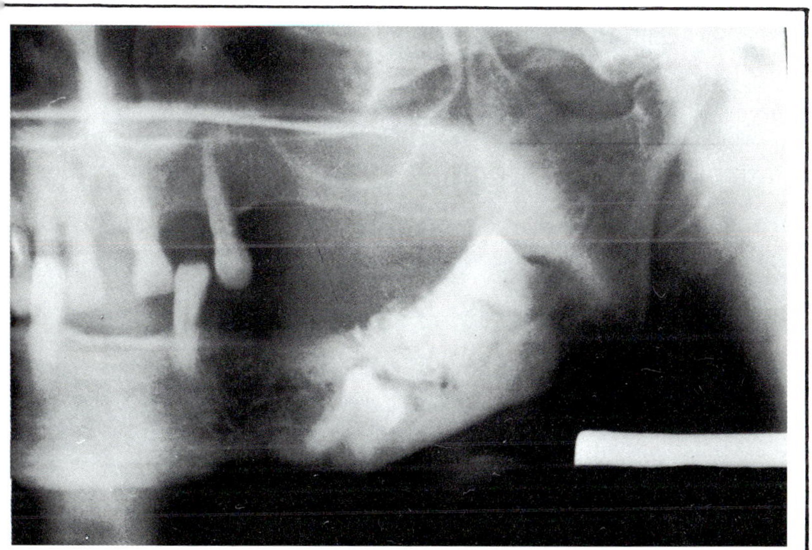

SECTION TEN: **WHITE PATCHES and ULCERS**

Fig. 246. A lesion of the floor of the mouth, white and wrinkled in nature, is an example of the non-hereditary variety of intra-oral epithelial naevus. *(750.86)*

Fig. 247. An aspirin burn of the labial sulcus and adjacent cheek; this is the usual site. *(N965)*

Fig. 248. Frictional keratosis of the right cheek along the occlusal plane of the teeth. *(528.6X)*

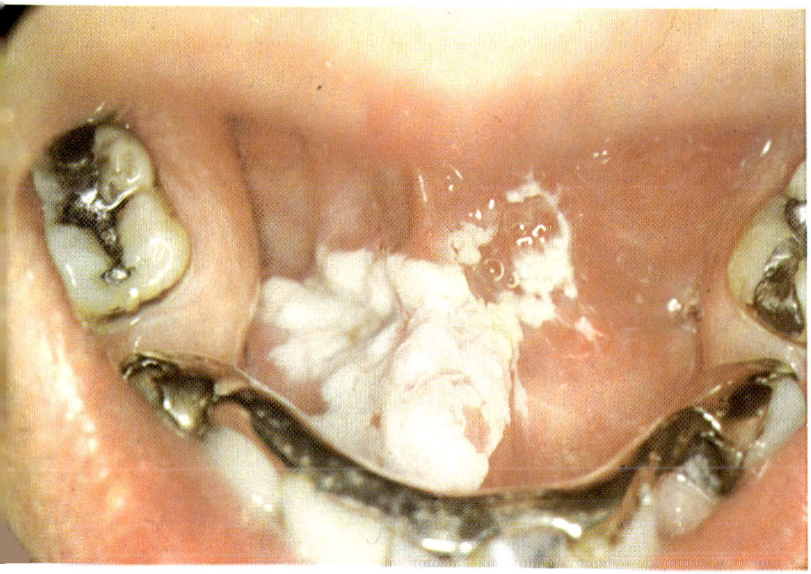

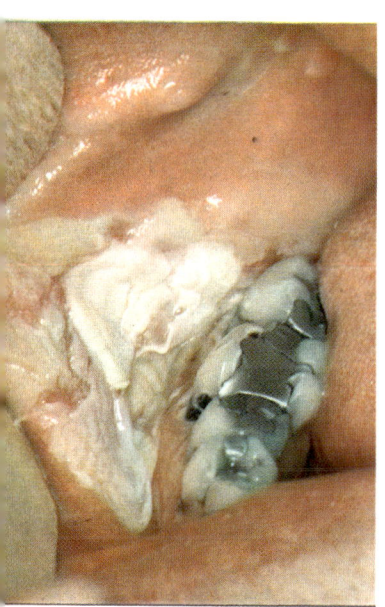
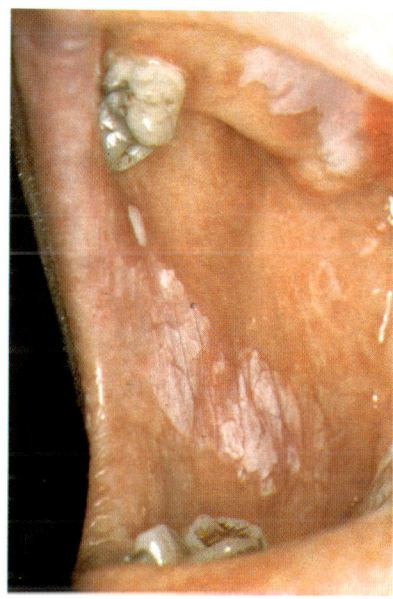

Fig. 249. The habit of tobacco-chewing is responsible for this lacy hyperkeratosis of the lower lip and gingival mucosa. Tobacco may be smoked, chewed or placed in the labial sulcus as snuff ("snuff-dipping"). All these habits lead to oral keratosis and predispose to oral carcinoma, especially if the patient also has some hepatic dysfunction. *(528.6X)*

Fig. 250. An area of lacy keratosis of the upper lip attributable to chlorpropamide medication which is commonly referred to as a lichenoid eruption. The other drugs which may precipitate such a reaction include amiphenazole, chlorothiazide, chloroquine, mepacrine and the heavy metals. *(N.977)*

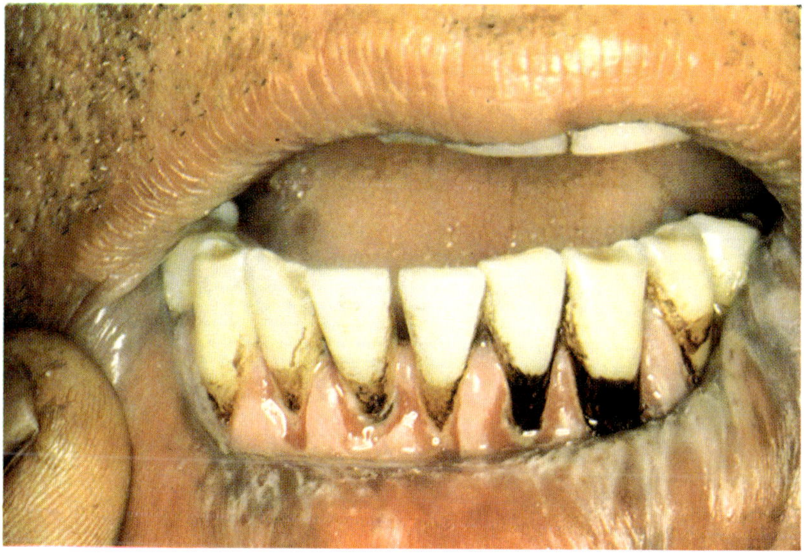

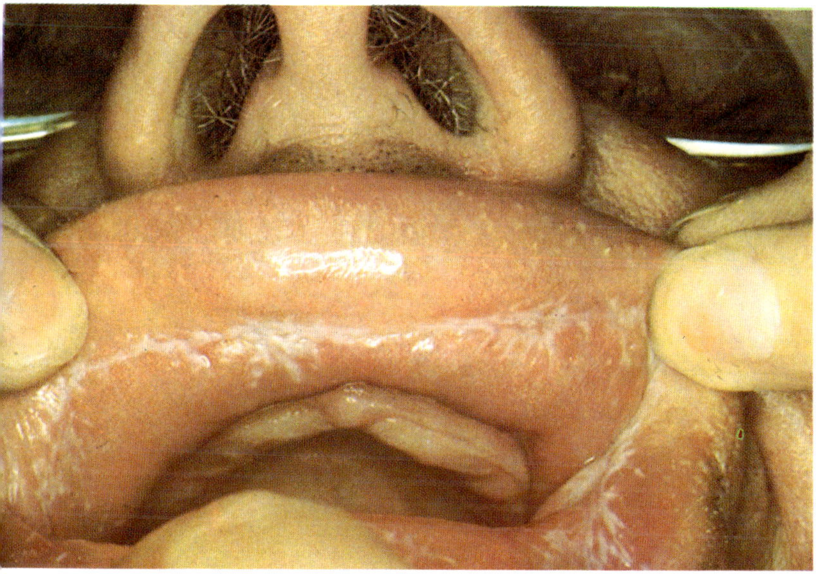

225

Fig. 251. This rather circinate hyperkeratosis of the buccal mucosa is due to lichen planus. *(697.08)*

Fig. 252. Another unusual form of lichen planus with extreme plaque-like hyperkeratosis. Lichen planus may present in many forms in the mouth but in most keratosis is a feature. Typically, mucosa of both cheeks adjacent to the molars is affected, but the tongue too is not infrequently involved. *(697.08)*

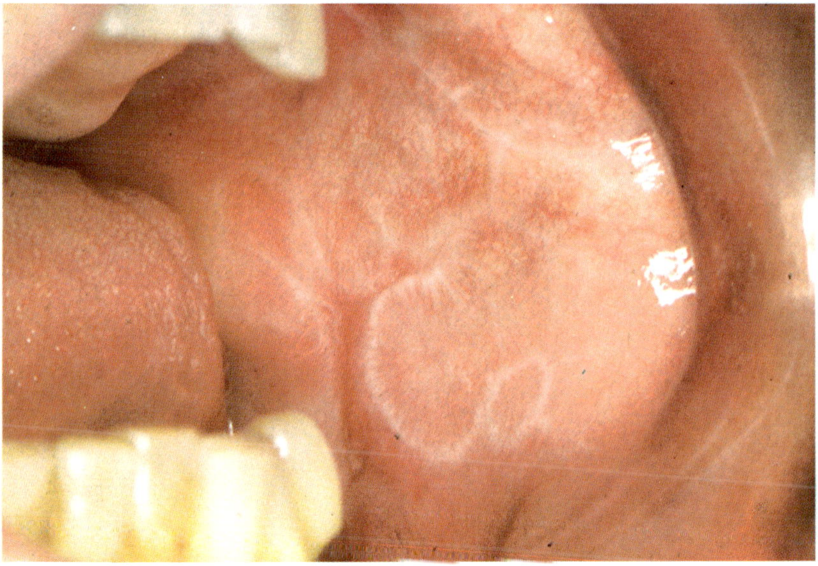

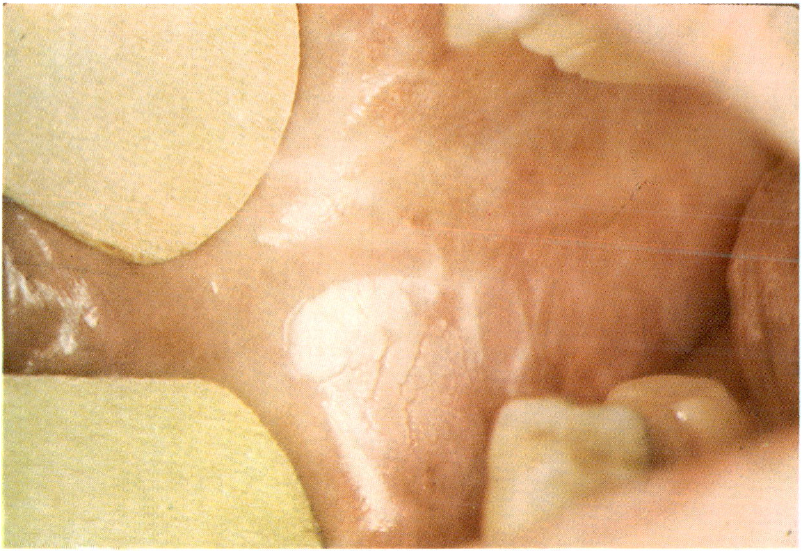

227

Figs. 253 & 254. An area of hyperkeratosis with ulceration in the area of the lingual fraenum. The underlying tissue feels hard since it consists of the genial tubercles together with the attached genioglossus muscles. The radiograph shows the extreme atrophy of the alveolus and the genial tubercles standing in the floor of the mouth. *(528.92)*

Fig. 255. Oral submucous fibrosis. Note the extra-articular ankylosis of the mandible due to the dense bands of fibrous tissue which tend to run vertically and eventually cause severe limitation of movement of the mandible. There is a strong predisposition to oral carcinoma in these patients. The disease is almost restricted to the peoples of the Indian sub-continent. *(528.8X)*

Fig. 256. Lichen planus of the tongue. *(697.08)*

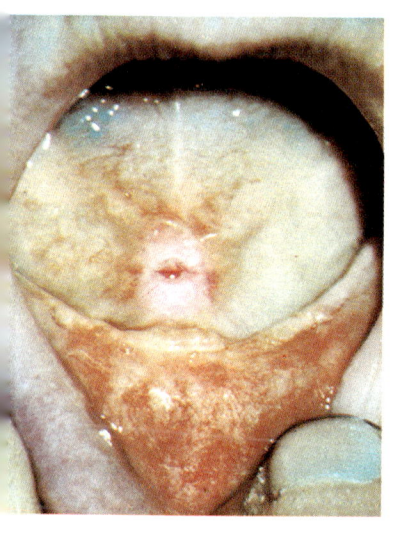
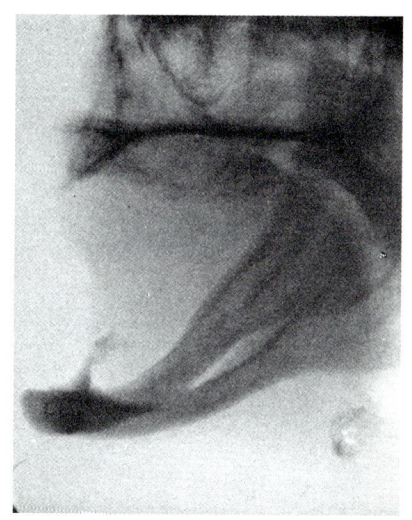
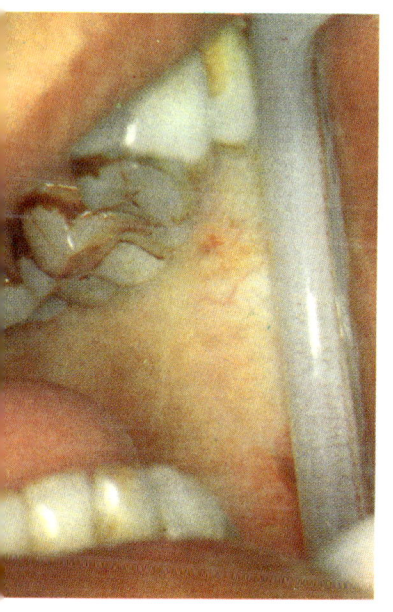
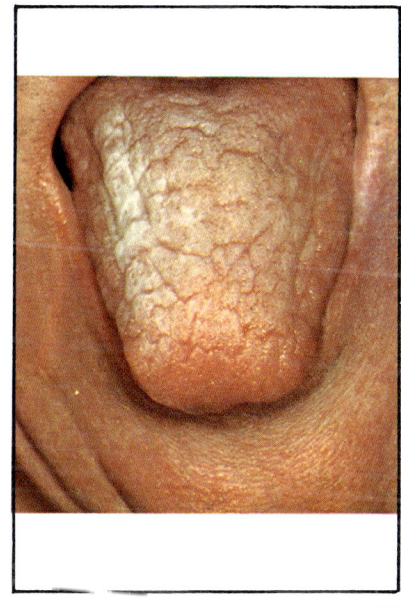

Fig. 257. White shaggy appearance of the tongue in a patient with uraemia due to chronic renal failure. The appearance is due to a coagulation of superficial protein by ammonia resulting from the degradation of salivary urea by oral bacteria. *(792.X0)*

Fig. 258. This is the appearance of the cheek in the same patient. Desquamation and ulceration may also occur and the mouth is sore, which may limit correct nutrition. *(792.X0)*

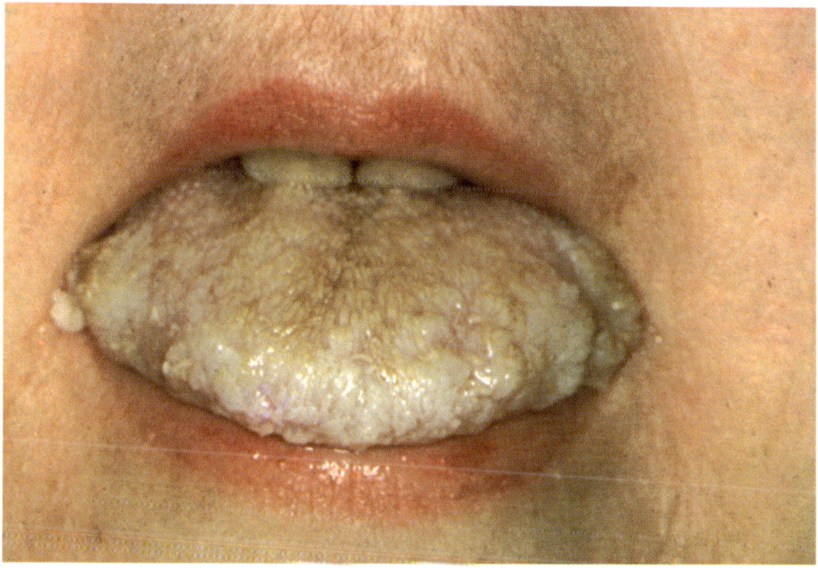

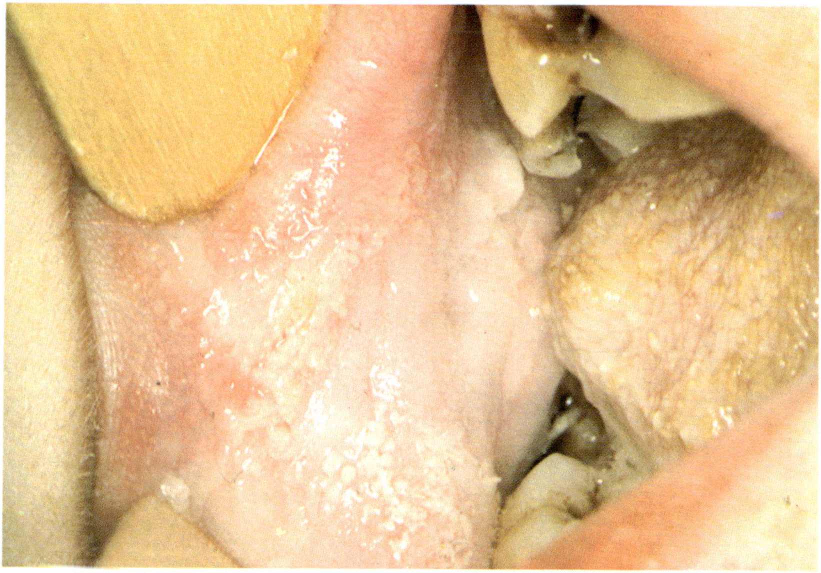

231

Fig. 259. A triangular hyperkeratotic plaque inside the commissure of the mouth is a form of hyperkeratosis due to chronic candidosis — Candidal leucoplakia. This is almost always associated with longstanding angular cheilitis. *(112.X9)*

Fig. 260. The typical appearances of cheek-biting seen in anxious people, usually young girls. There is part hyperkeratosis and part loss of epithelium due to nibbling of the cheek. *(528.93)*

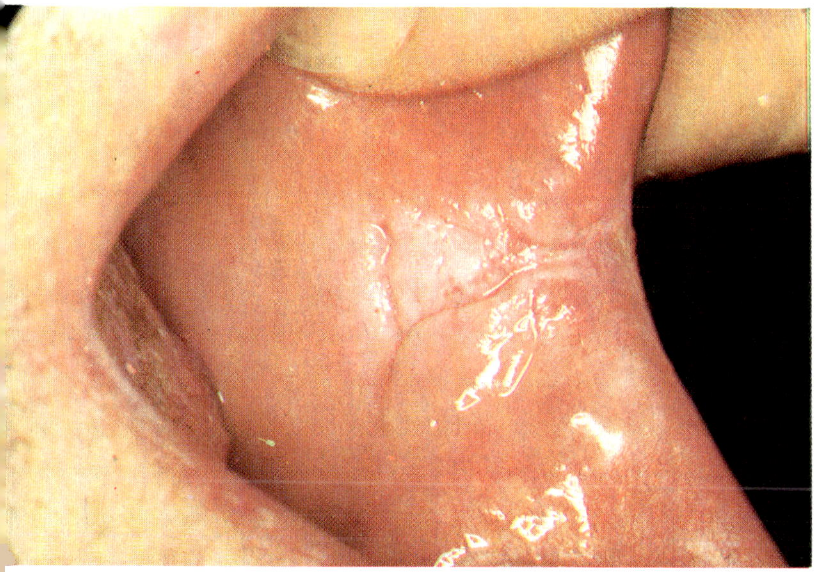

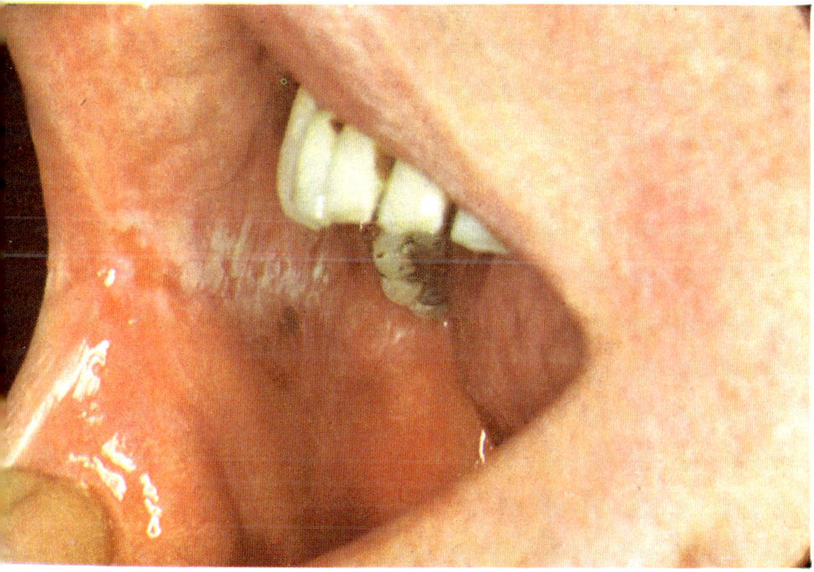

233

Fig. 261. This small white papilliferous plaque is a squamous-cell carcinoma — even a simple white patch may be a neoplasm. *(144.XX)*

Fig. 262. A further example of a very early carcinoma of the mandibular alveolus. *(143.1X)*

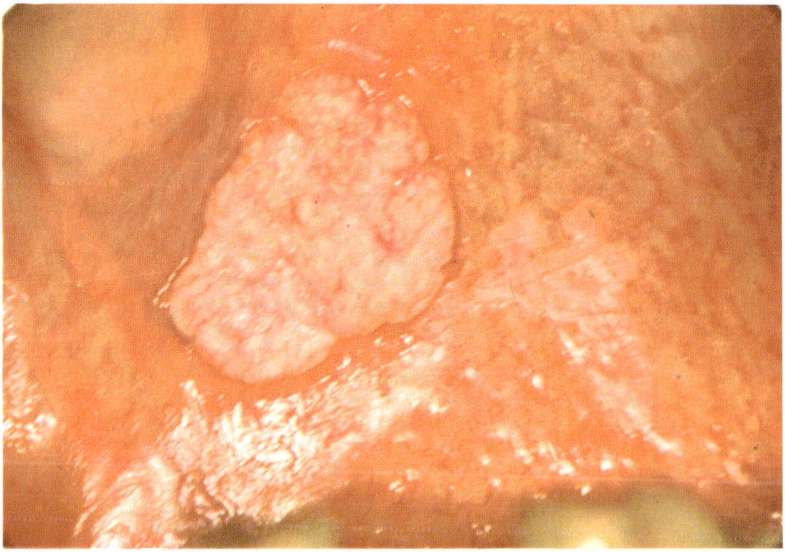

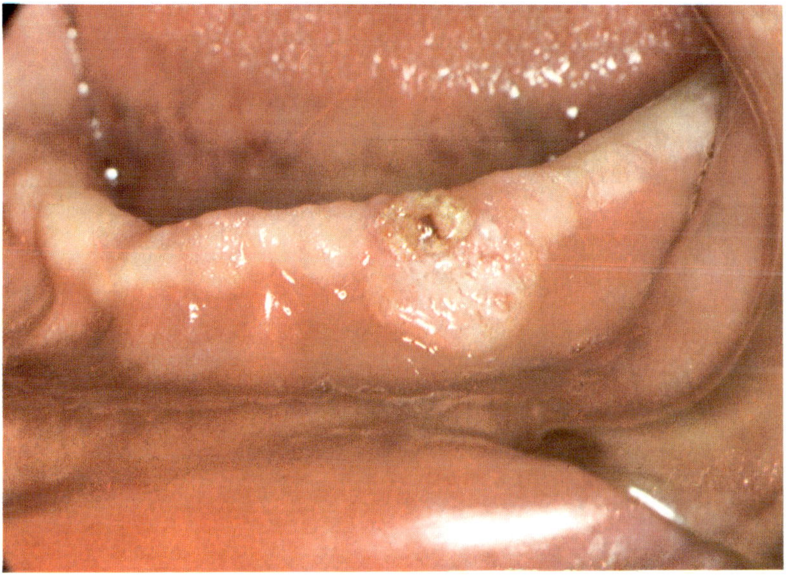

235

Fig. 263. Aphthae appear as here in crops which recur at irregular intervals. They occur consistently on the non-attached (non-keratinised) oral mucosa, and very rarely form on the hard palate, attached gingiva or dorsum of the tongue. *(528.20)*

Fig. 264. These white plaques on the tongue represent fibrinous exudate covering ulcers. This is an example of Behçet's syndrome with associated genital ulceration and recurrent iritis. *(136.X1)*

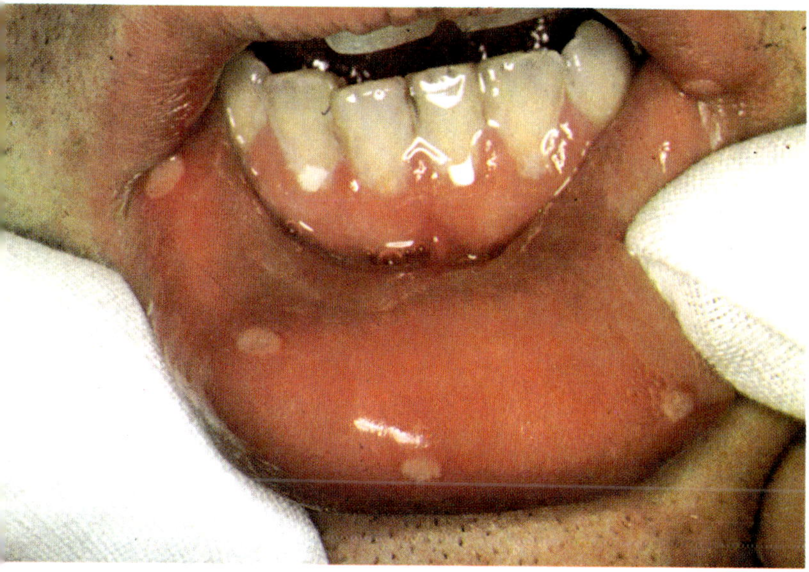

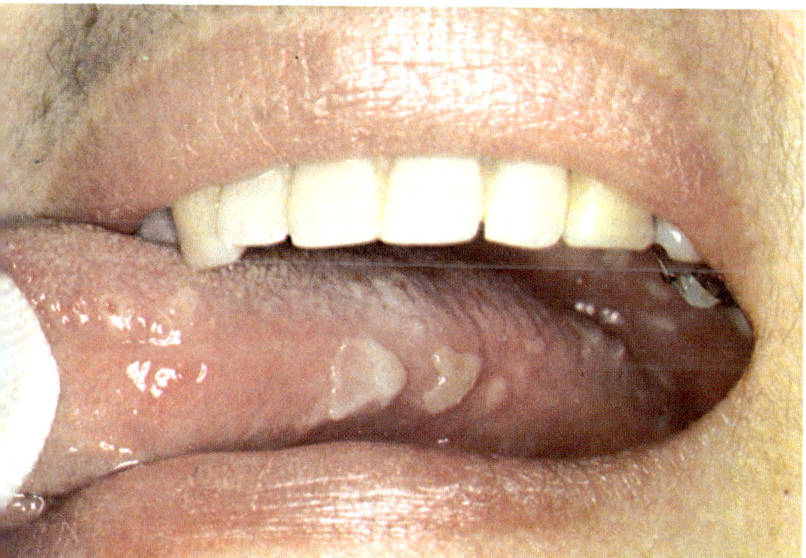

237

Fig. 265. An aphthous ulcer. Note its oval shape, gently shelving floor and inflamed, rampart-like periphery. *(528.20)*

Fig. 266. More aphthous ulcers, but in an unusual situation on the soft palate.

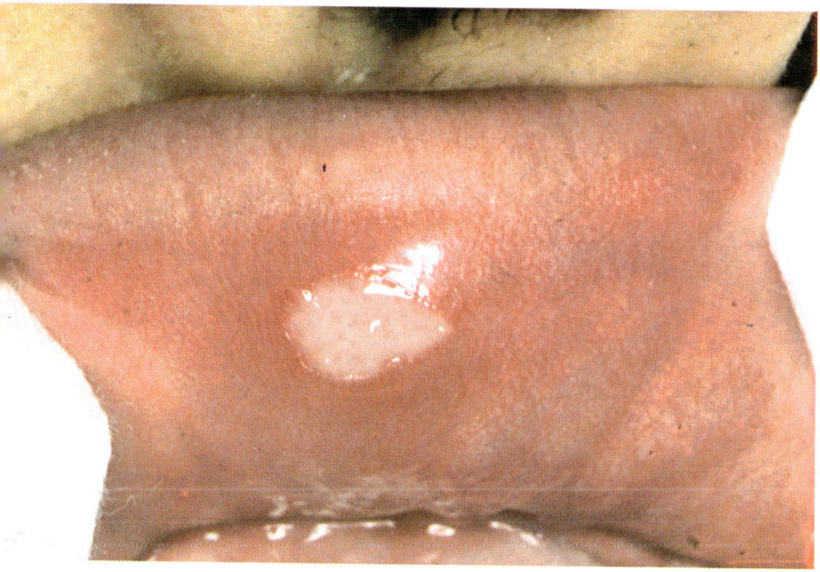

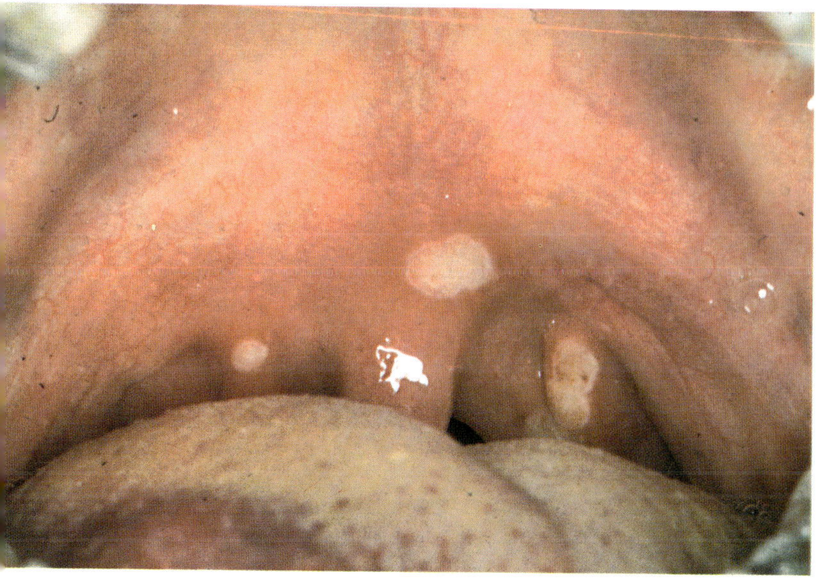

239

Fig. 267. This white patch of the tongue was of unknown aetiology and biopsy confirmed hyperkeratosis. The condition is labelled idiopathic keratosis or leucoplakia. *(529.72)*

Fig. 268. Herpetiform aphthae constitute a variant of recurrent aphthae which may be of viral aetiology but are not related to herpetic infection. A multitude of tiny ulcers develop usually on the cheeks or floor of the mouth and some may coalesce to form large irregular lesions. They are characteristically associated with widespread erythema. Herpetiform ulcers may occur in the mouth in Behçet's syndrome. *(528.20)*

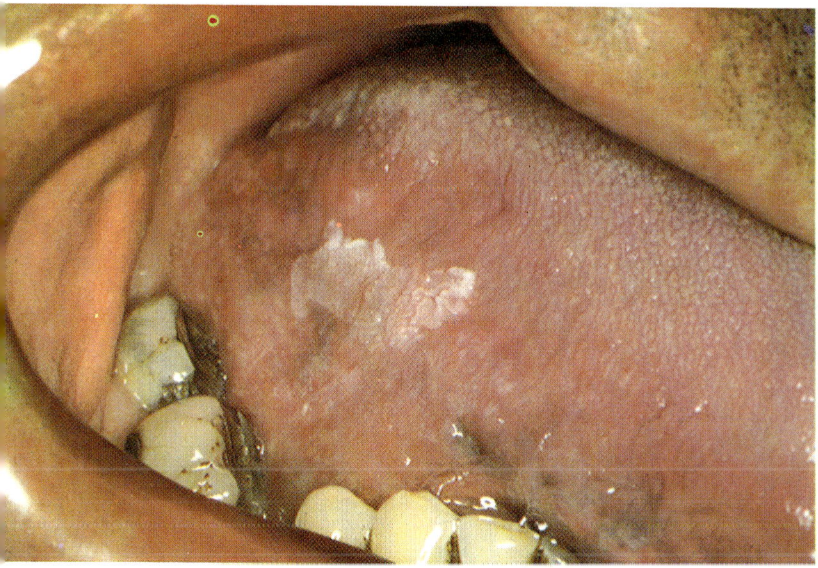

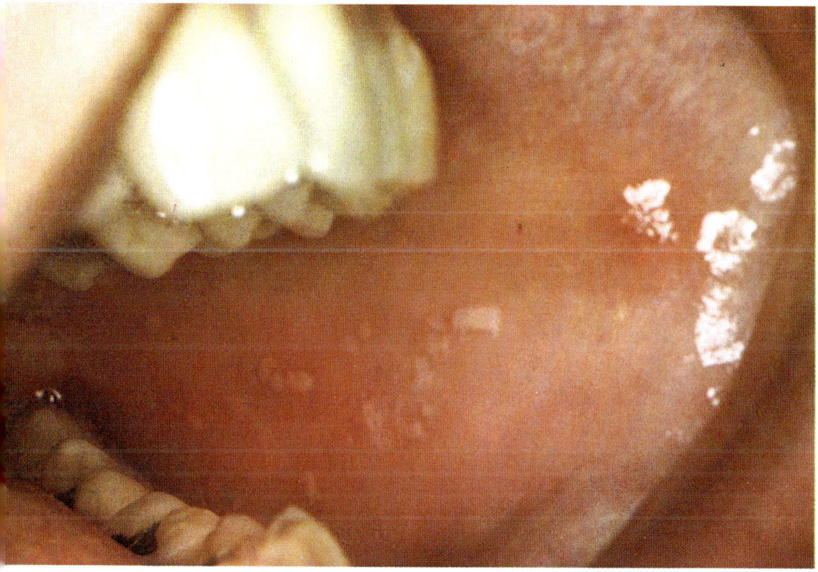

Fig. 269. Large irregular ulcers with fibrinous exudate which proved to be the remains of the intra-epithelial bullae of pemphigus. In any recurrent oral ulceration it is important to search for evidence of previous bullae, especially if there is not much surrounding inflammation. All vesiculo-bullous lesions in the mouth, except those obviously due to primary herpes, require biopsy. *(694.X0)*

Fig. 270. Pemphigus vulgaris again — the bullous nature of the cheek lesion is here clearly visible. The oral lesions of pemphigus are prominent and may antedate cutaneous involvement. Early diagnosis is vital and requires biopsy and examination for acantholytic cells. The bullae of pemphigus are superficial, fragile and can be made to extend readily by gentle friction (Nikolsky's sign).

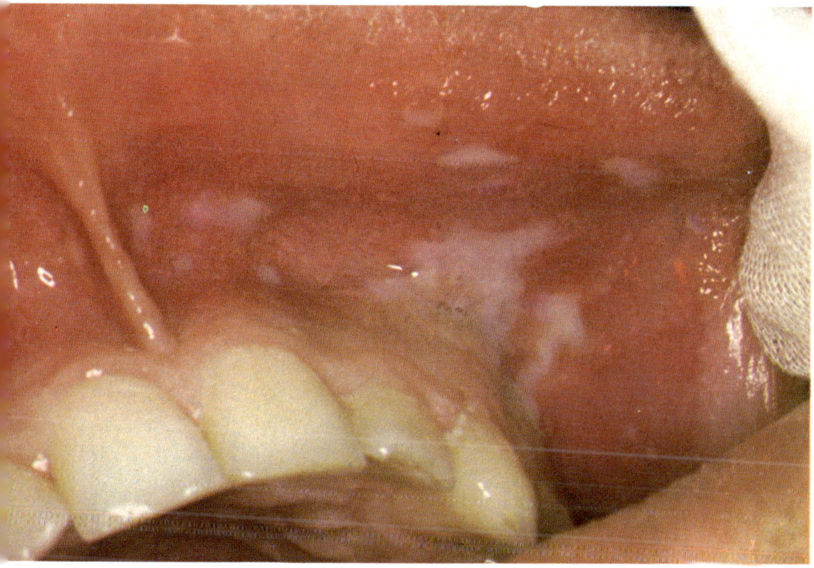

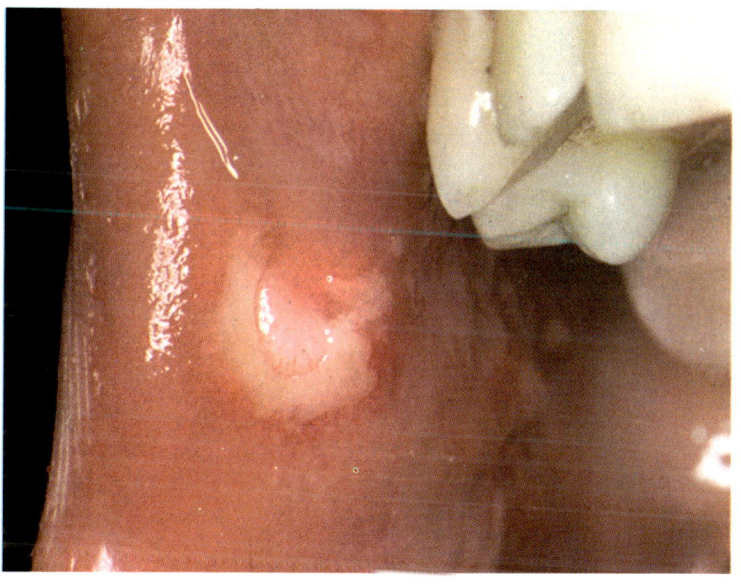

Fig. 271. Primary herpes simplex of the finger, which was associated with oral lesions in a case of extensive primary infection. *(054.X9)*

Fig. 272. Primary herpes simplex in an adult showing ulcers on the gingivae and palate. Vesicles are also present. *(054.X1)*

Fig. 273. Primary herpes simplex in childhood. The disease is seen at its most florid in young children but, unfortunately, it is difficult with patients at that age to photograph the oral eruption successfully. The vesicular stage is transient but it is unusual to see a case without vesicles. These occur particularly on the attached mucosa. *(054.X1)*

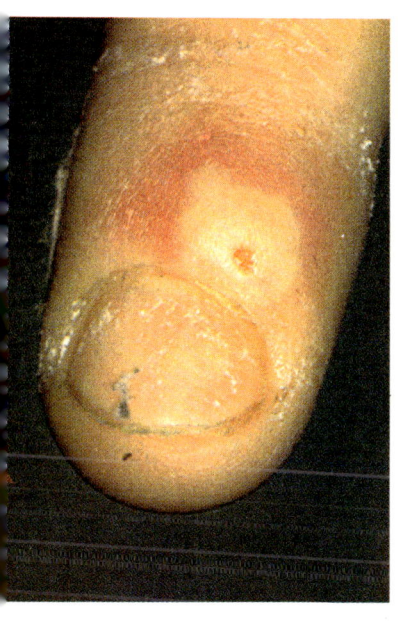
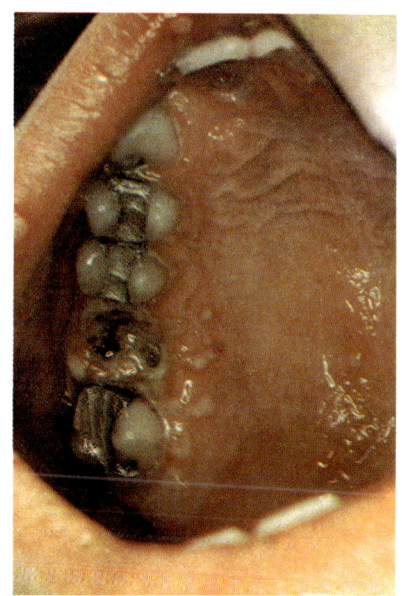

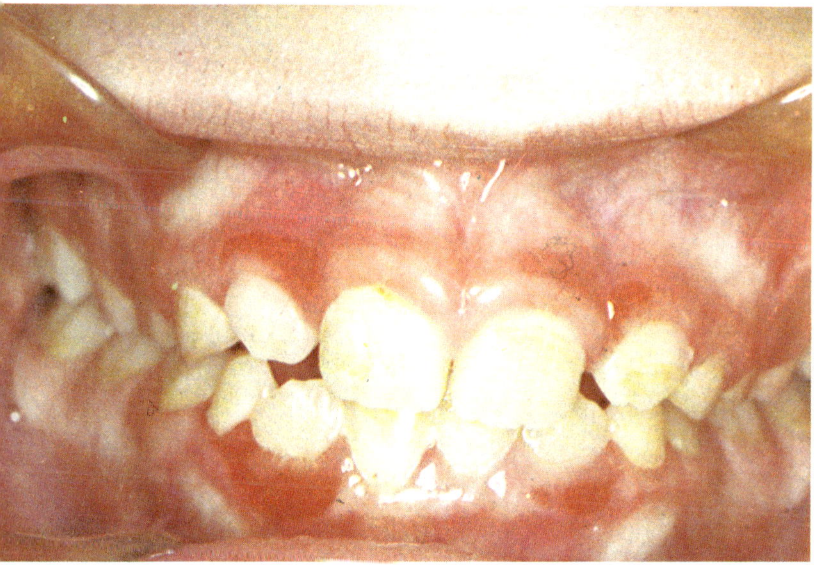

Fig. 274. A traumatic ulcer of the lower lip. Note the loss of the maxillary left central incisor. *(528.92)*

Fig. 275. A traumatic ulcer with a blood-stained base at the hard/soft palate junction due to irritation by a denture. *(528.92)*

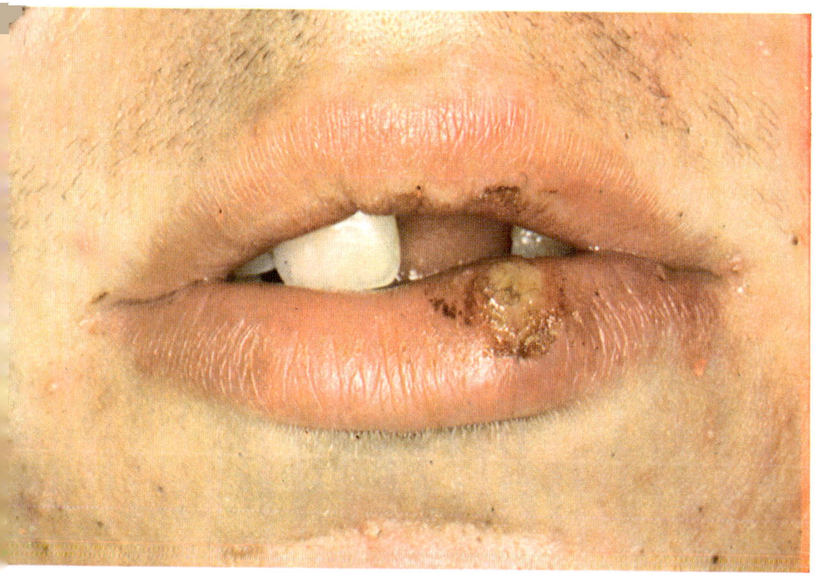

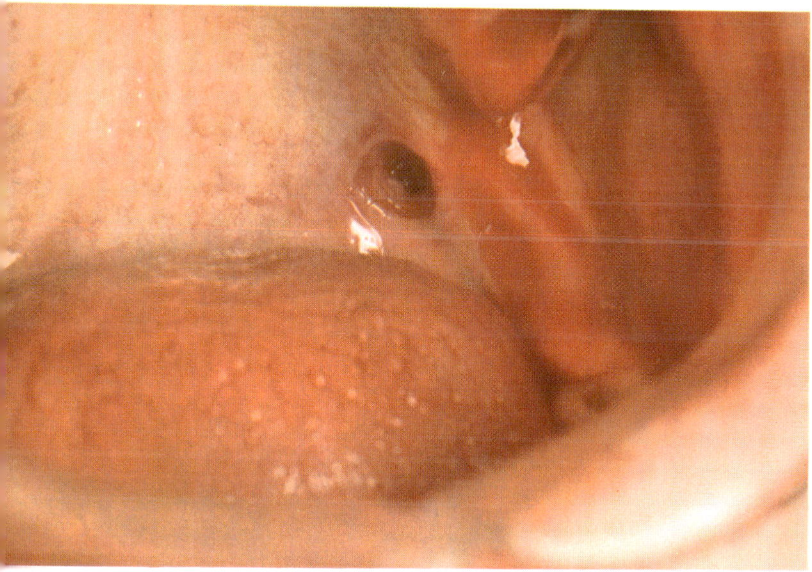

247

Fig. 276. Extensive diffuse inflammation with patchy ulceration typical of erythema multiforme. Note the blood crusting on the lip. *(695.10)*

Fig. 277. Here is an extensive area of erosion and ulceration of the cheek due to discoid lupus erythematosus. Cutaneous lesions were well marked. *(695.40)*

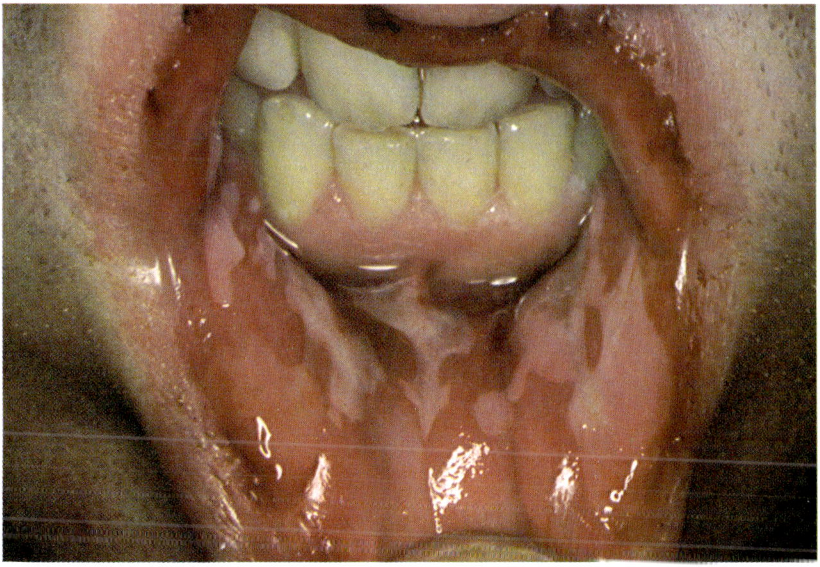

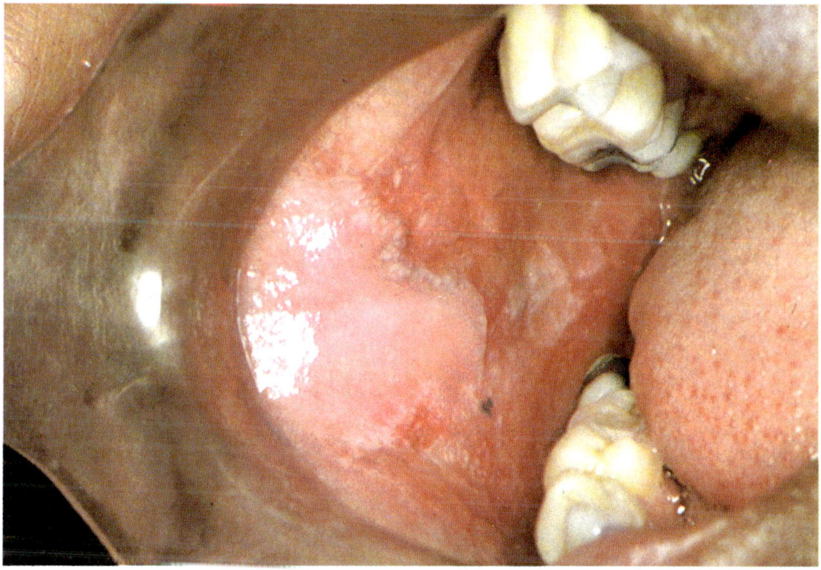

249

Fig. 278. Another example of erythema multiforme with central vesiculation. *(695.10)*

Fig. 279. Extensive patchy inflammation and ulceration — again of erythema multiforme. This oral eruption develops rapidly with irregular inflammation, vesiculation and ulceration. The gross involvement of the lips is typical. There may be cutaneous or other mucosal lesions.

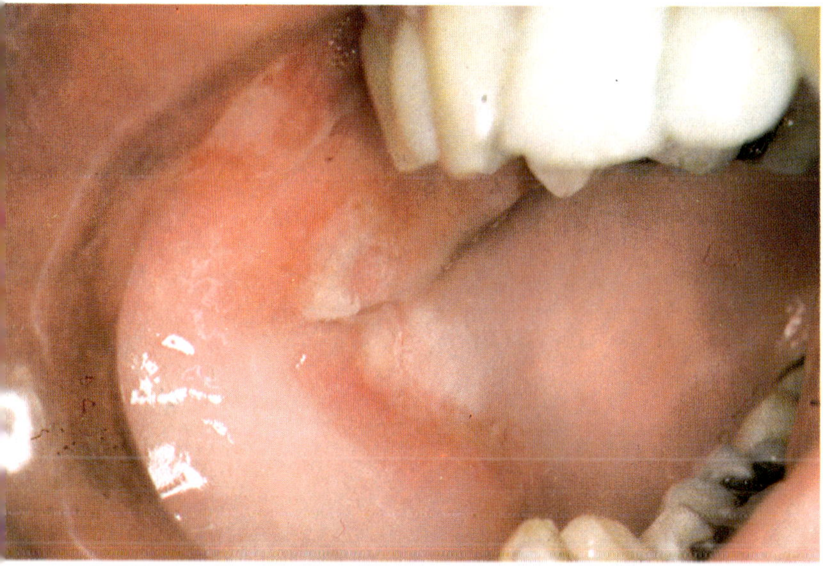

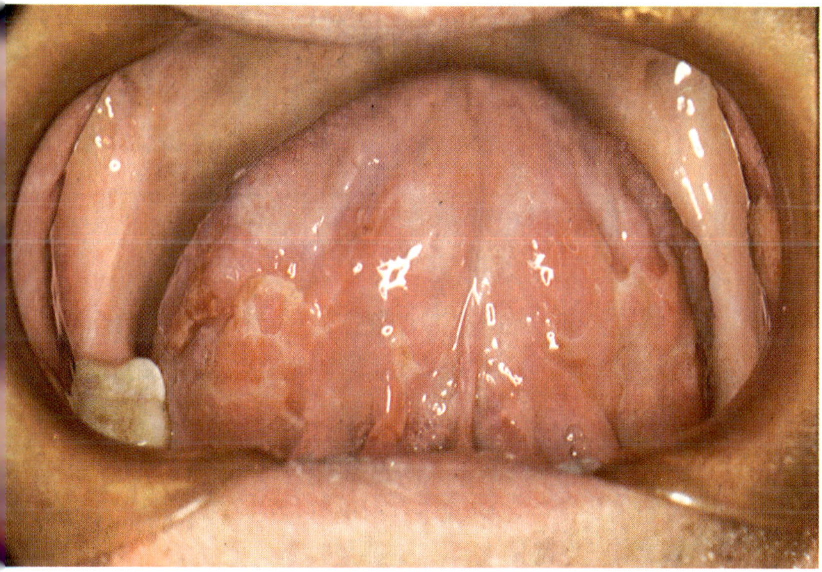

251

Fig. 280. This bullous lesion — typically without surrounding inflammation — is due to pemphigus. *(694.X0)*

Fig. 281. This widespread lacy erythema with associated ulceration is erosive lichen planus. *(697.01)*

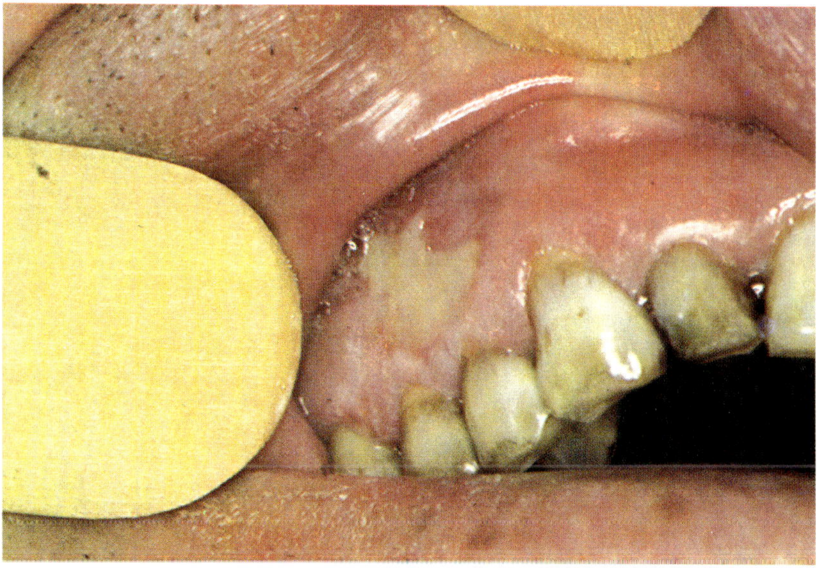

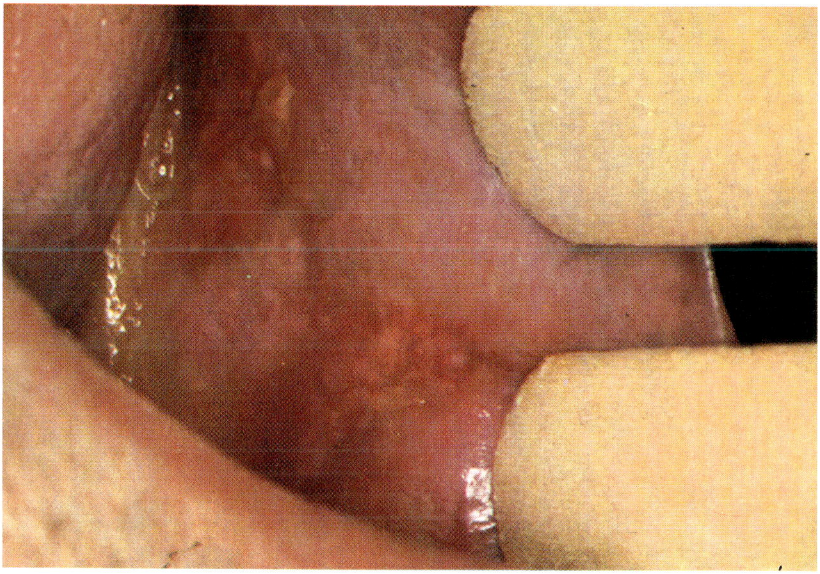

253

Fig. 282. Hand, foot and mouth disease — the cutaneous lesions. This disease is due to Coxsackie A virus and remits rapidly. The oral lesions are transient. *(074.90)*

Fig. 283. Pemphigus vulgaris showing the large flaccid bullae. *(694.X0)*

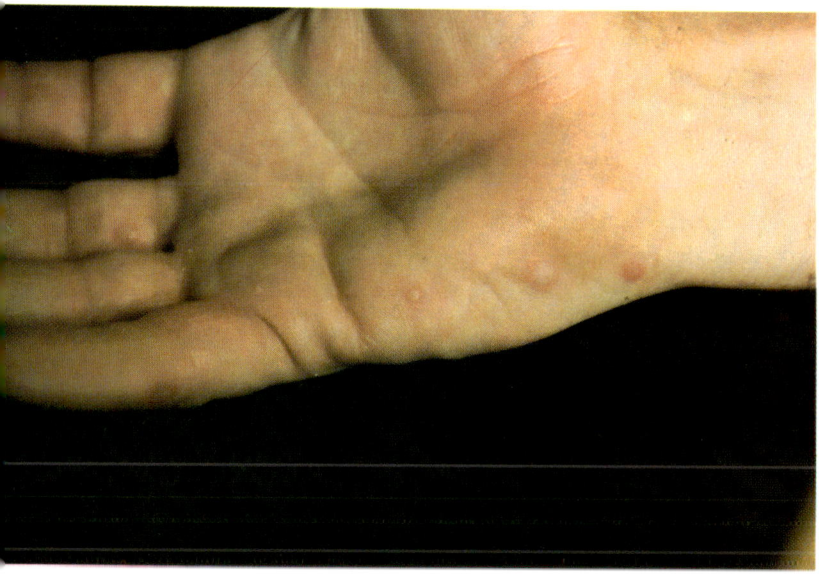

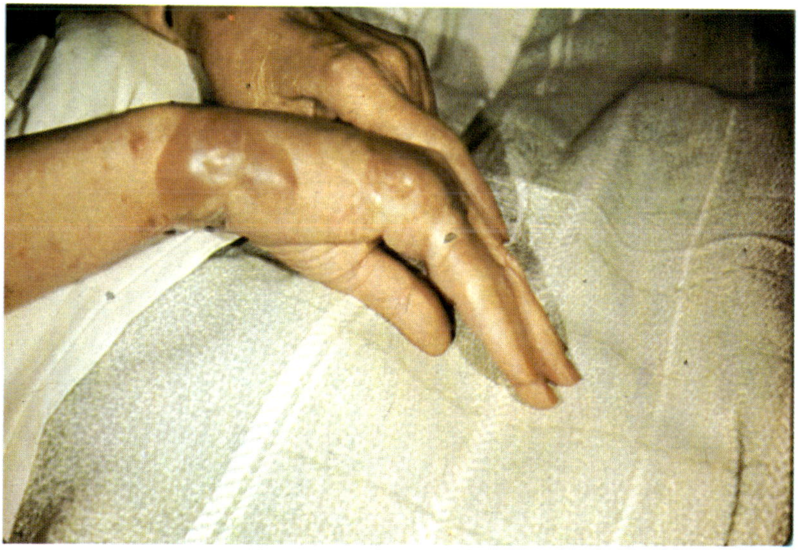

255

Fig. 284. Neuropathic ulcer of the upper alveolus. The patient was completely anaesthetic in the distribution of the right maxillary nerve following an alcohol injection for trigeminal neuralgia. The upper right lateral incisor — loosened by the trauma which originally provoked the ulcer — subsequently fell out. *(N.997)*

Fig. 285. Extensive macerated ulceration of the lower right third molar region due to fusospirochaetal infection. The infection may spread forward as typical ulcerative gingivitis. *(101.X1)*

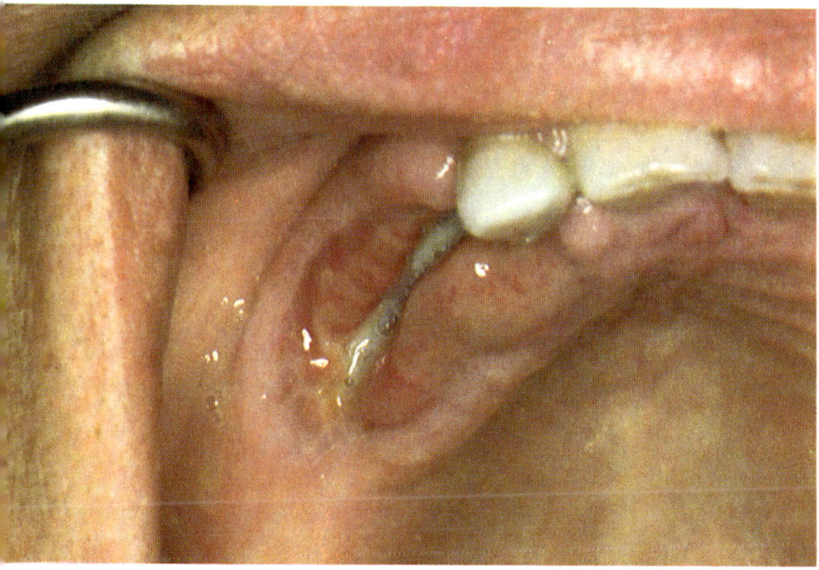

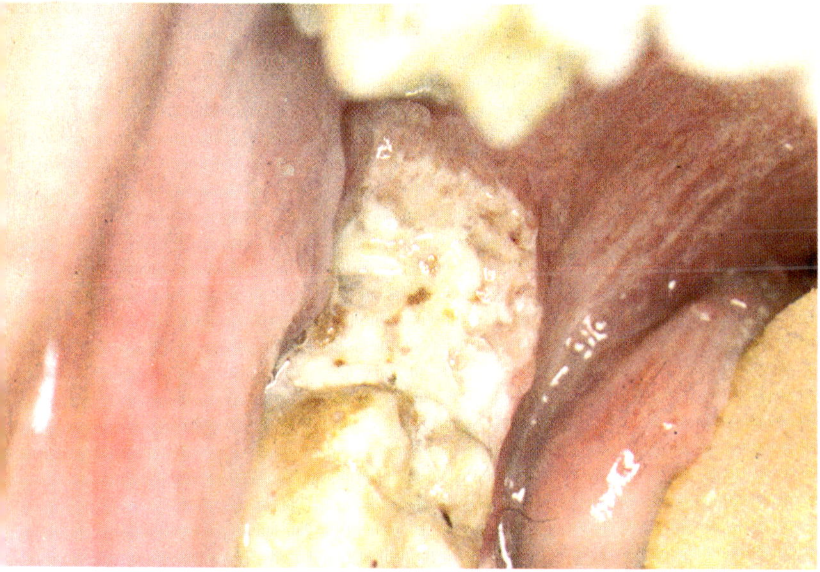

257

Fig. 286. An ulcer of the gingival margin due to arsenic having leaked from the pulp chamber of the lower left first molar through a proximal cavity. (Fortunately, the use of arsenic has now been almost entirely abandoned.) *(N.985,1)*

Fig. 287. Massive ulcer of the upper alveolus following extraction of teeth with gross periodontal disease. This ulcer is another expression of local fusospirochaetal infection. *(101.X1)*

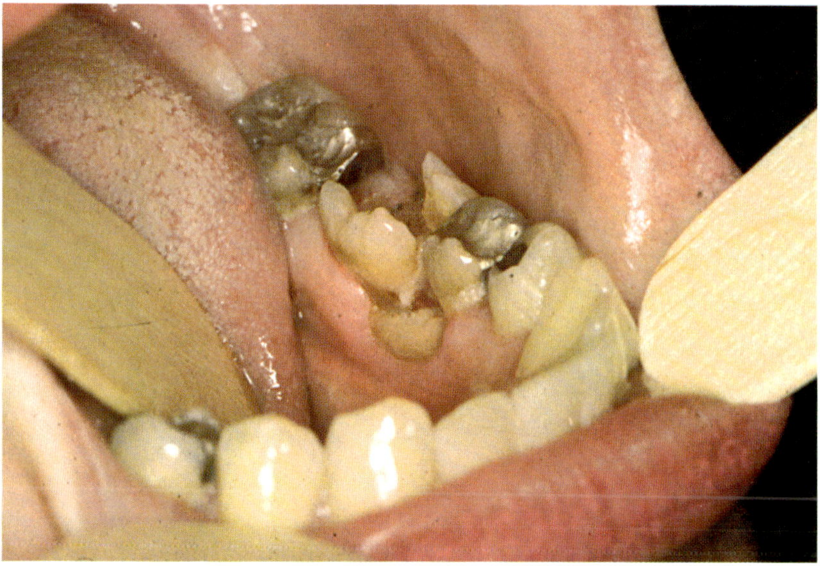

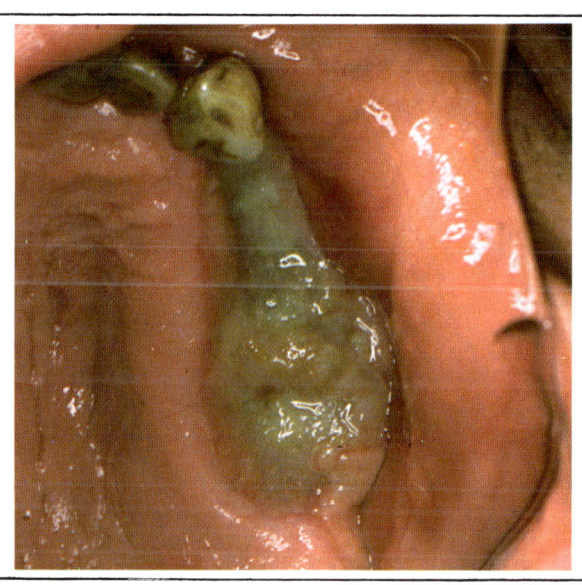

SECTION ELEVEN: **JAW DEFORMITIES**

Figs. 288, 289, 290 & 291. Hypoplasia of structures derived from the first branchial arch on the left. The face is asymmetrical due to unilateral mandibular hypoplasia.
Fig. 289. Shows the malformed left ear. The intra-oral view **(Fig. 290)** shows the disordered occlusion due to the left mandibular hypoplasia, and this is also confirmed by the x-ray. *(524.04)*

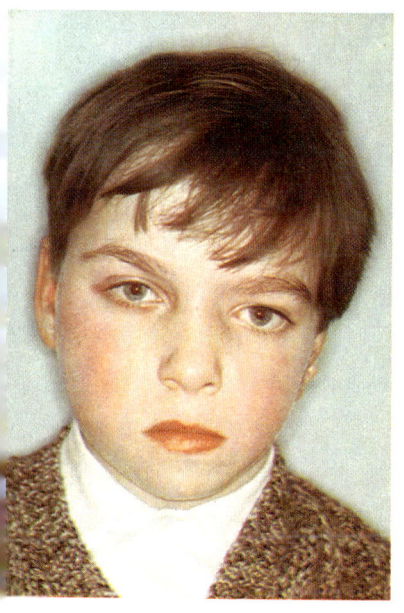
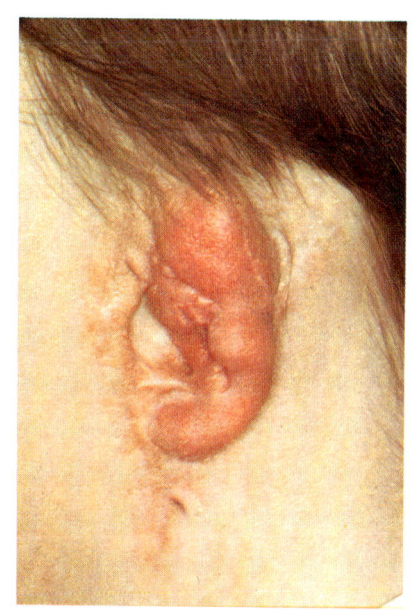
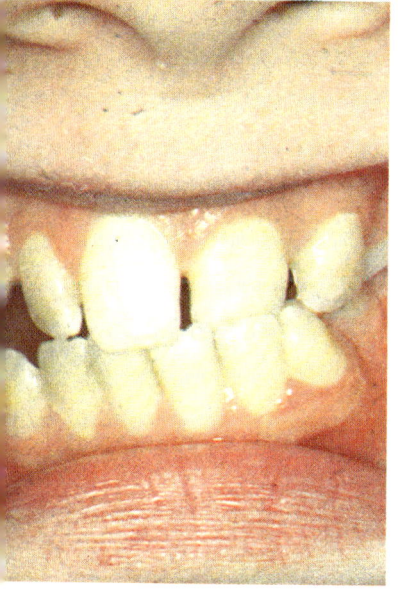
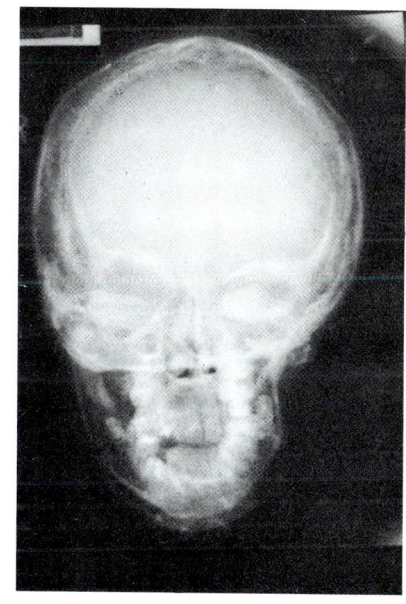

201

Figs. 292 & 293. Another case of the "first arch syndrome", this time right-sided. *(524.04)*

Fig. 294. The x-ray of the affected side shows the markedly shortened ascending ramus of the jaw with a small condyle and coronoid process. Compare this with the normal side, **Fig. 295.**

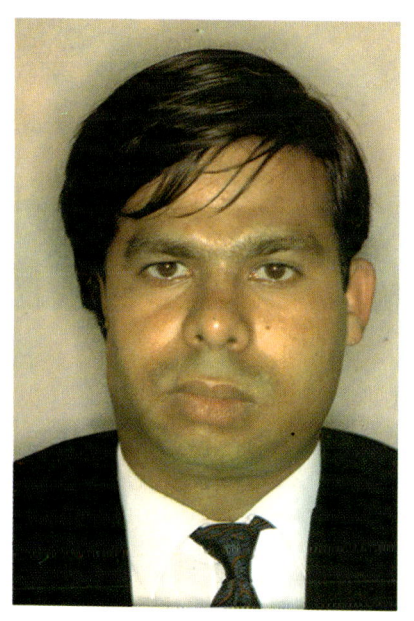
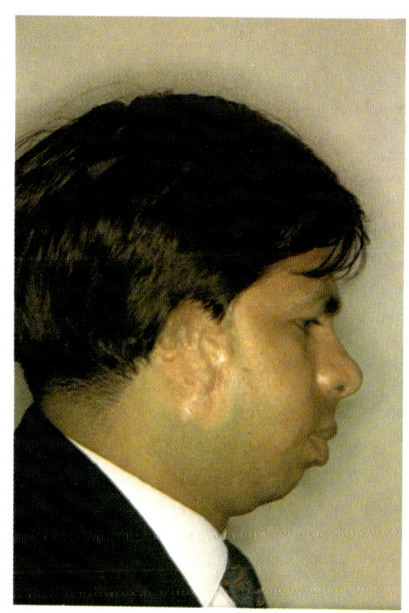
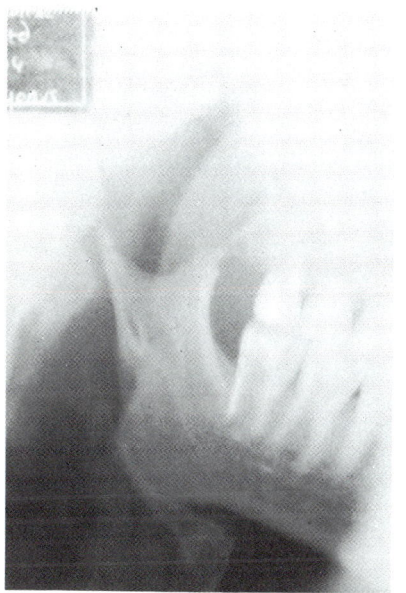
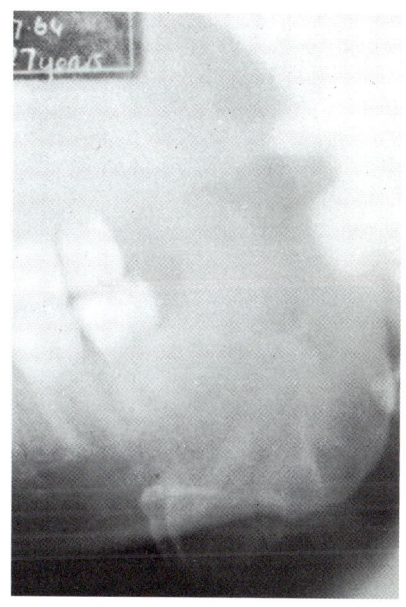

Figs. 296 & 297. Idiopathic condylar hyperplasia (R). In this condition the condylar growth centre is overactive and there are two clinical subdivisions. In one, as here, the ascending ramus is lengthened and the lower border is bowed down with the chin point deviated to the opposite side. The intra-oral view shows normal occlusion on the left with an open bite on the right. *(729.X0)*

Figs. 298 & 299. The x-rays show the considerable increase in the height of the right ascending ramus. In the lateral view the remarkable downward bowing of the lower border is clearly seen. The second variety is characterised by a displacement of the mandible to the opposite side with less vertical distortion of the mandible.

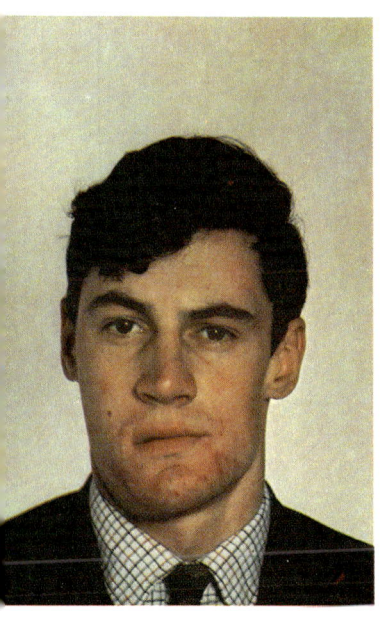
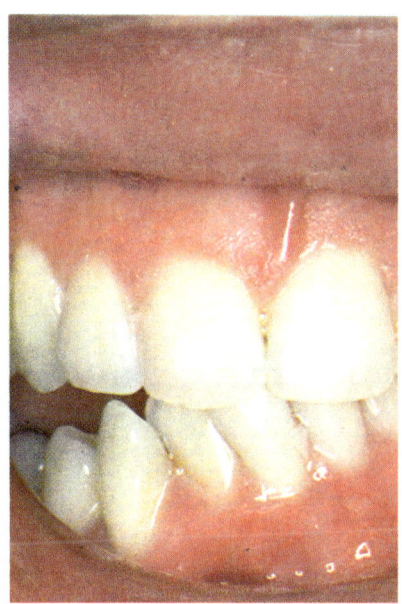
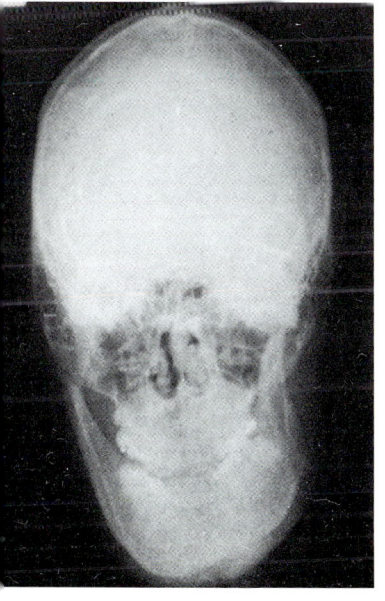
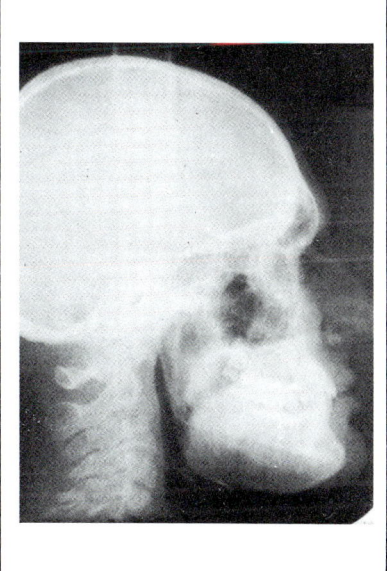

Fig. 300. Right masseteric hypertrophy, which is a condition of unknown aetiology and may be bilateral.

Fig. 301. Absence of muscles of mastication on the right side — aetiology unknown.

Fig. 302. Atrophy of muscles of mastication on the right side following poliomyelitis some years before. The x-ray **(fig. 303)** shows the poorly developed right angle of the mandible.

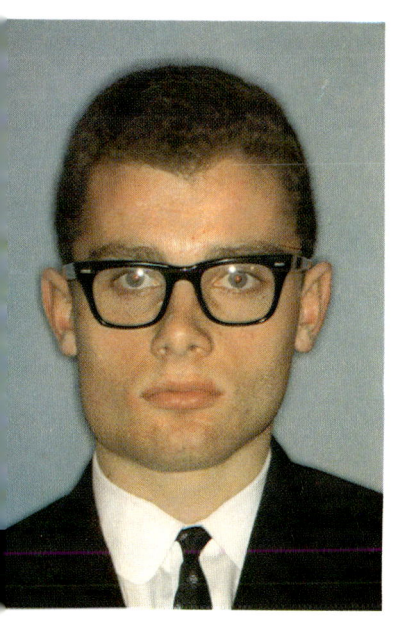
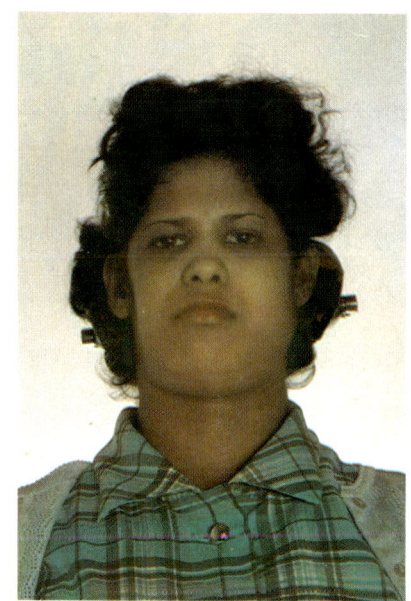
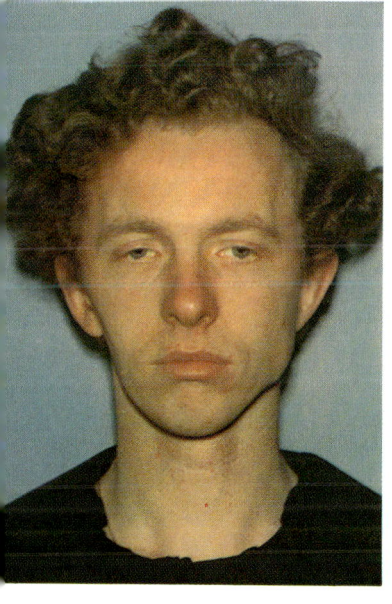
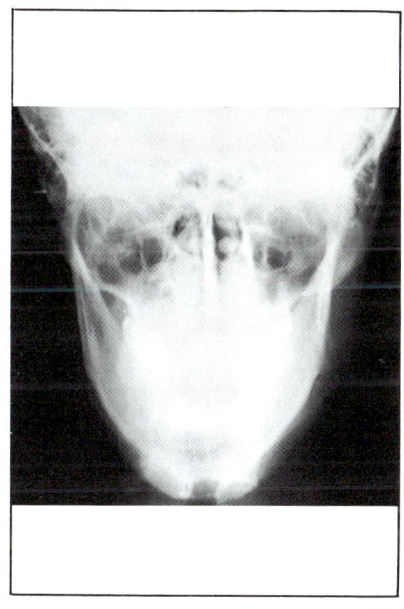

Fig. 304. This patient has facial asymmetry due to displacement of the mandible to the right. The condition developed gradually over the preceding 10 years. Note the occlusal disharmony with the mandible displaced one unit to the right **(fig. 306)**. The x-ray **(fig. 305)** reveals an osteochondroma of the left condyle. *(213.X0)*

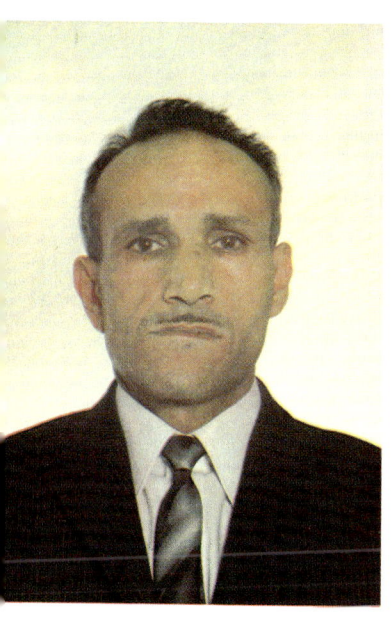
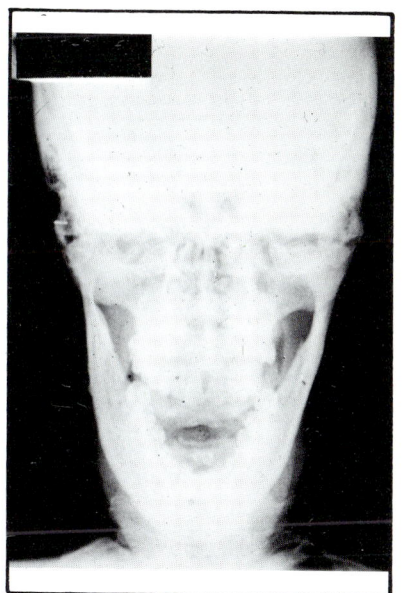

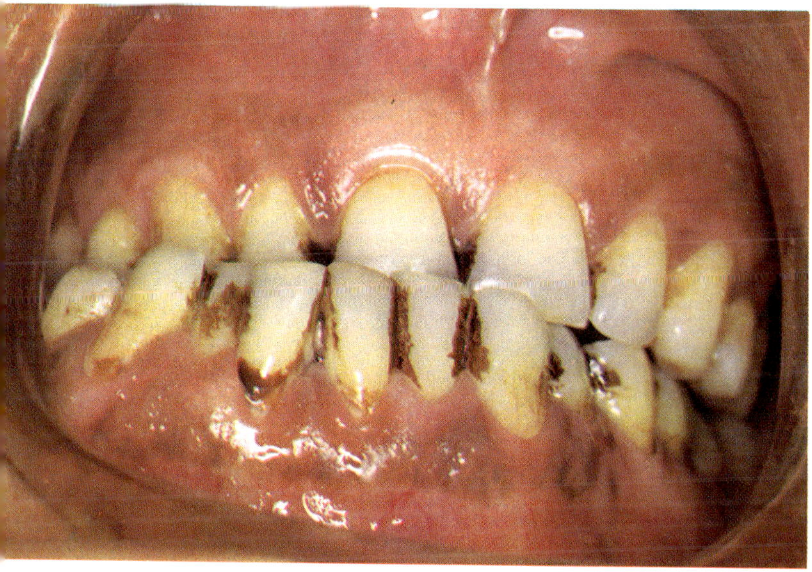

Figs. 307, 308, 309 & 310. Bird-face deformity due to reduced growth at the condylar centres leading to mandibular hypoplasia. The recession of the chin point and narrowing of the mandible are typical. The intra-oral view shows gross malocclusion with secondary crowding and narrowing of the maxillary anterior segment. The x-ray shows the relatively short basal bone of the mandible with a short ascending ramus and a high Frankfort mandibular plane angle. The angle of the mandible projects, and this is a result of appositional growth in response to the masseter and medial pterygoid muscle insertions which leads to a typical antegonial notch. *(524.04)*

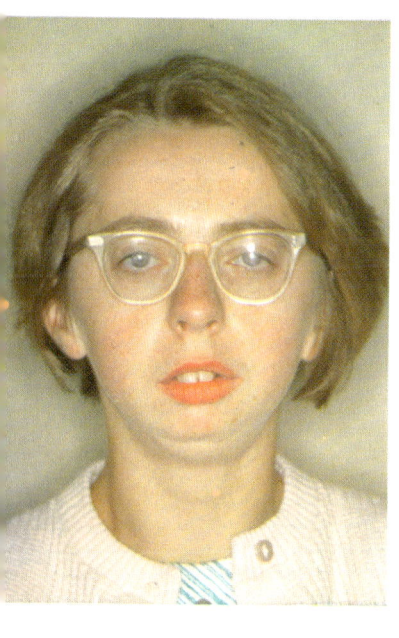
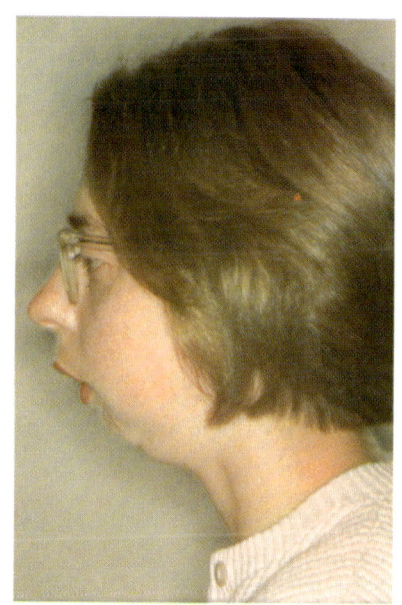
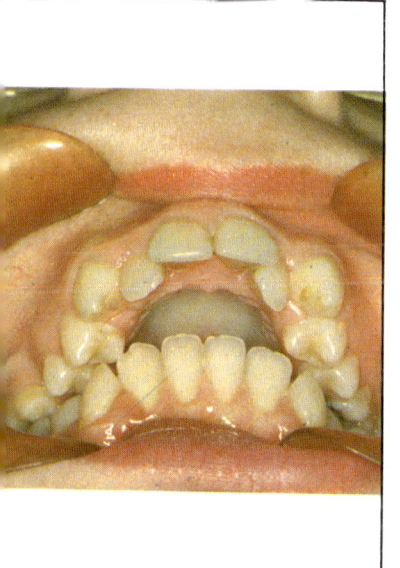
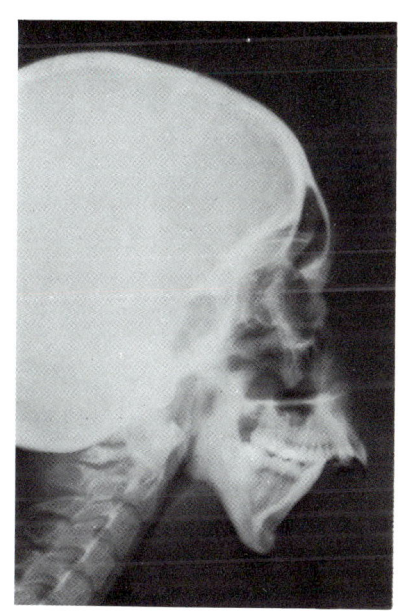

271

Fig. 311. Anterior open bite extending only from the premolar regions with increased proclination of the upper incisors. The posterior occlusion is normal. *(524.24)*

Fig. 312. The x-ray reveals that the skeletal abnormality is limited to the premaxillary region.

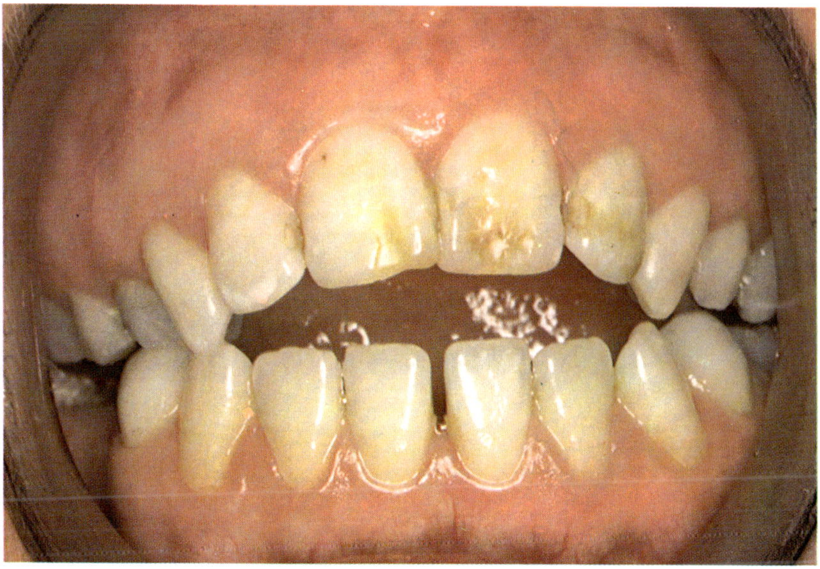

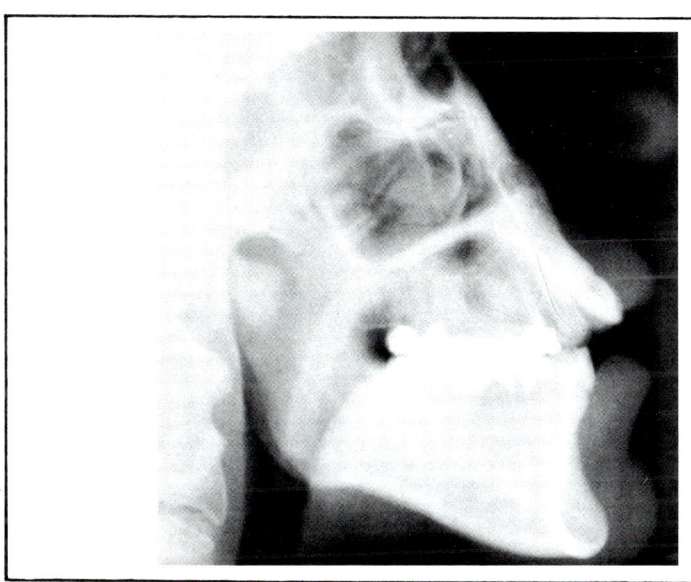

Fig. 313. Anterior open bite, but here the only tooth contact is between the upper and lower second molars with a progressively increasing discrepancy between the teeth. Such a type of open bite is referred to as the "skeletal variety". There was no history of trauma, and the patient had not experienced any difficulty in eating. *(524.24)*

Fig. 314. The x-ray reveals the normal configuration of maxilla and mandible and their lack of conformity. *(524.24)*

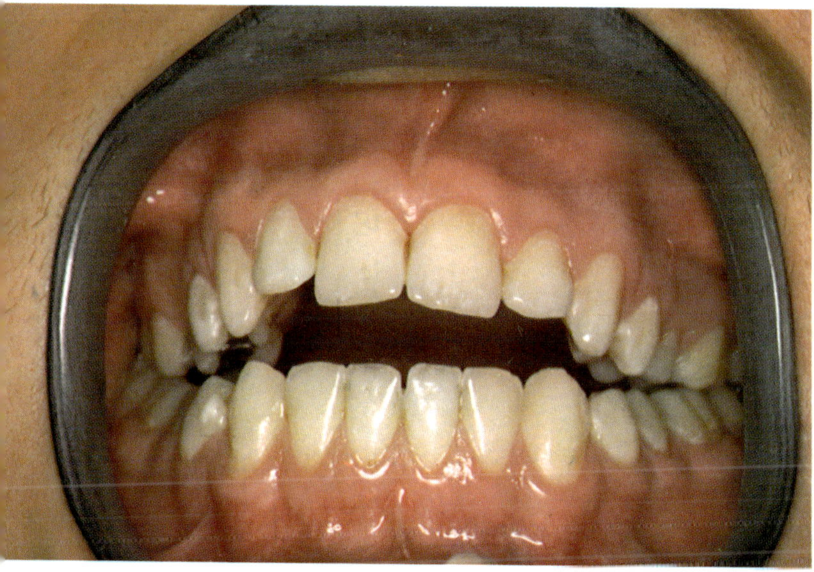

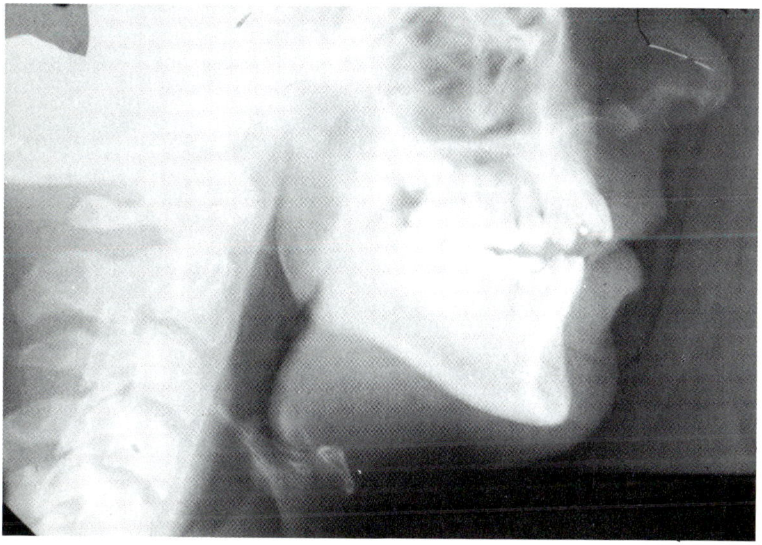

275

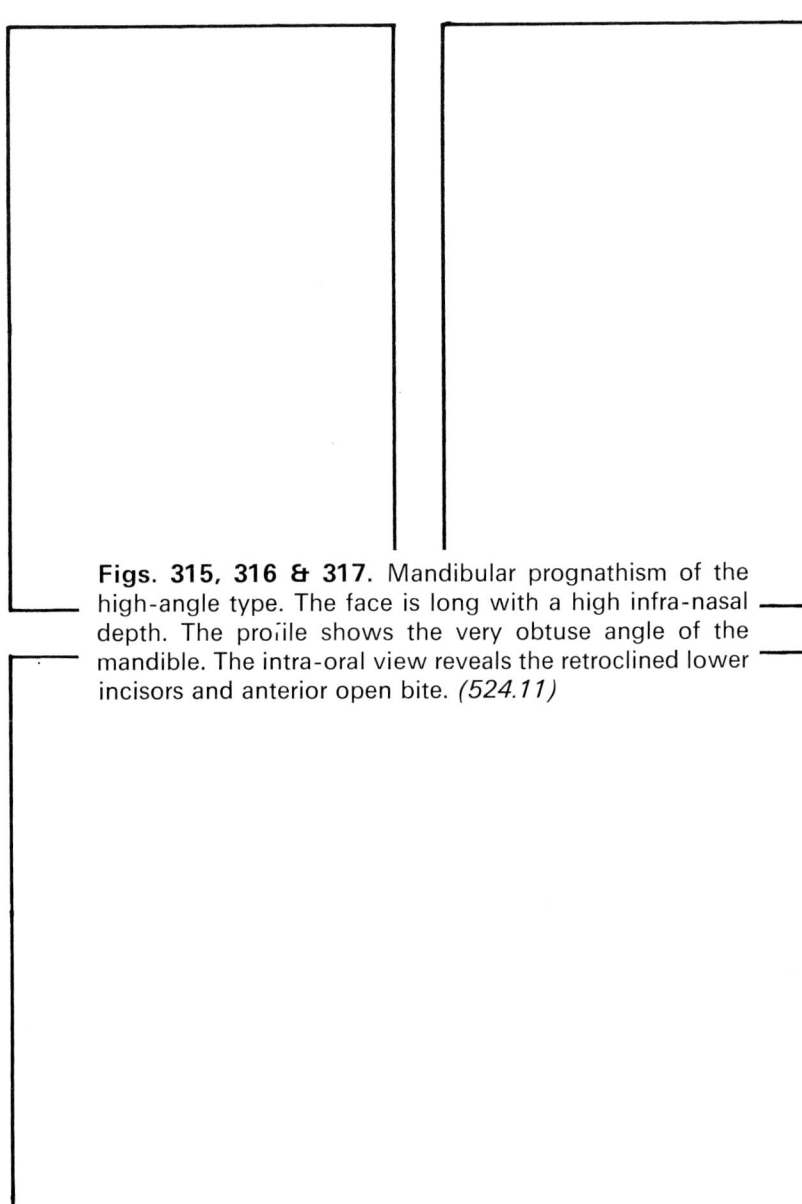

Figs. 315, 316 & 317. Mandibular prognathism of the high-angle type. The face is long with a high infra-nasal depth. The profile shows the very obtuse angle of the mandible. The intra-oral view reveals the retroclined lower incisors and anterior open bite. *(524.11)*

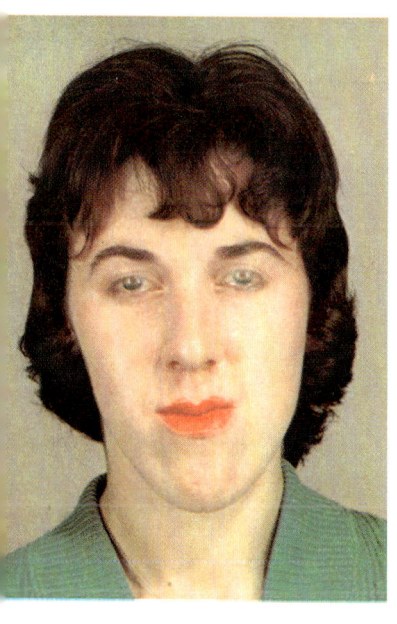
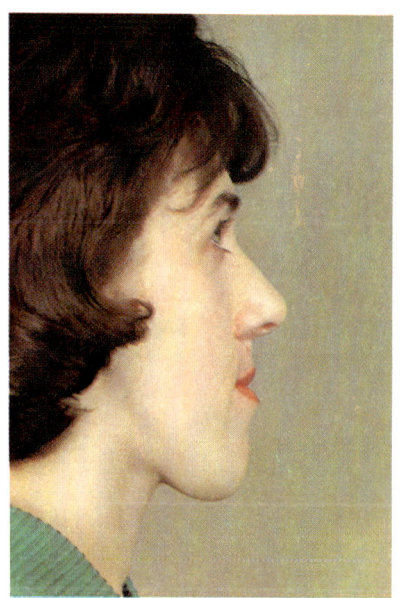

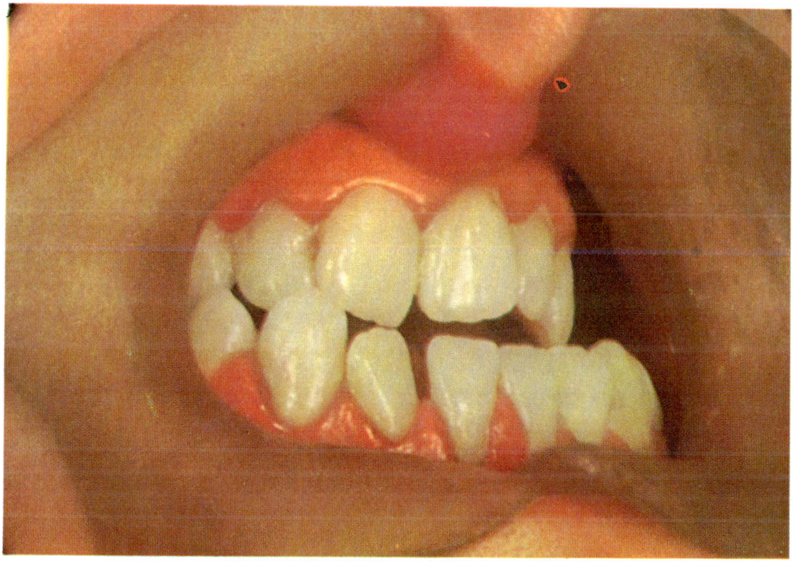

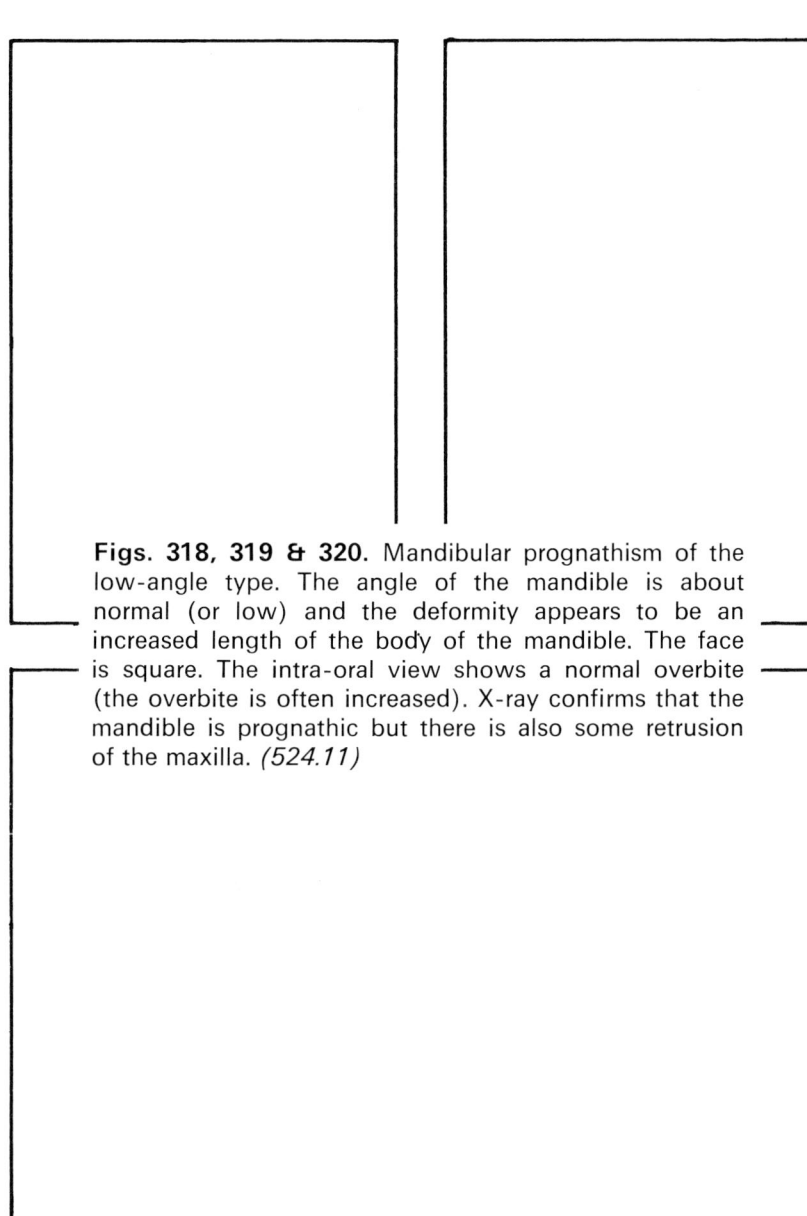

Figs. 318, 319 & 320. Mandibular prognathism of the low-angle type. The angle of the mandible is about normal (or low) and the deformity appears to be an increased length of the body of the mandible. The face is square. The intra-oral view shows a normal overbite (the overbite is often increased). X-ray confirms that the mandible is prognathic but there is also some retrusion of the maxilla. *(524.11)*

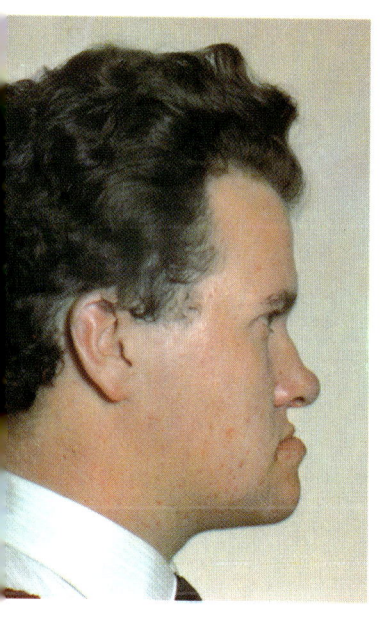
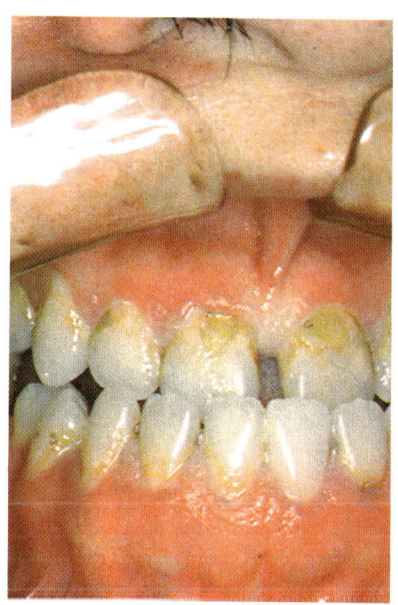
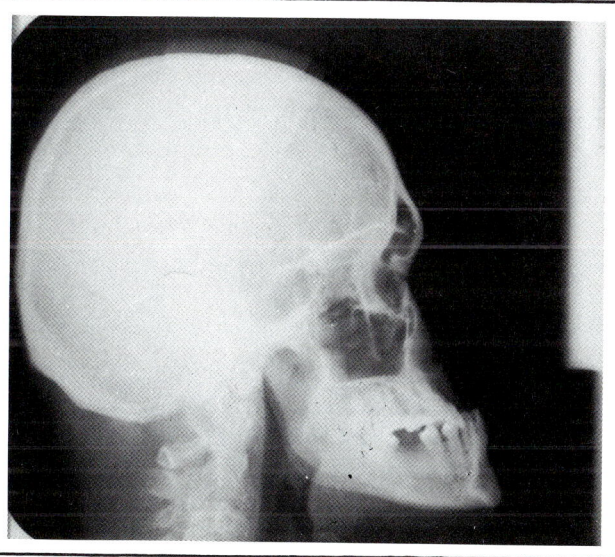

Fig. 321. Bilateral "dislocation" of the temporomandibular joints. The patient is unable to close the mouth. The condition is due to muscle spasm when the mouth is fully open. *(N830.01)*

Fig. 322. An attempted tooth extraction which resulted in gross loss of soft-tissue and fracture of the mandible. *(N802.31; N997)*

Figs. 323 & 324. The Reverse Towne's and lateral oblique projections show the line of fracture in the right third molar region and the retained tooth roots.

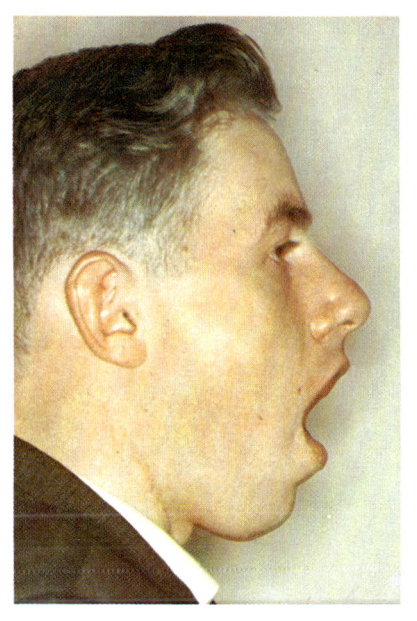
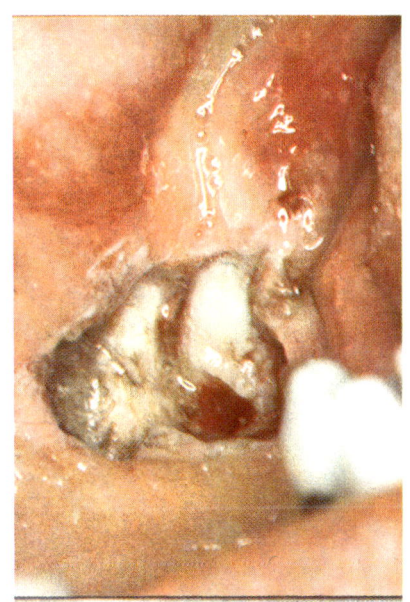
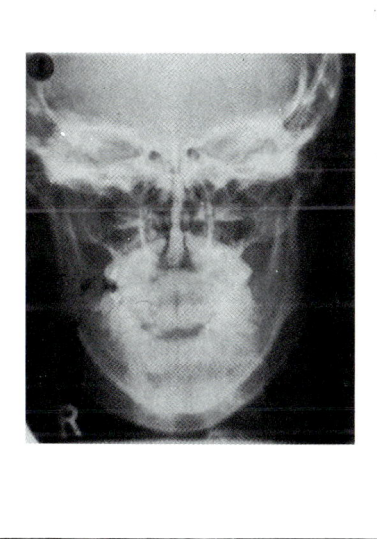
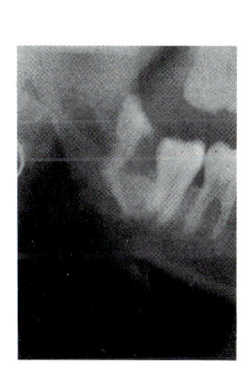

Fig. 325. A fracture of the mandible between the lower left lateral incisor and lower left canine with obvious occlusal derangement. *(N802.31)*

Fig. 326. Fracture of the left zygomatic arch showing a typical depression of the skin of the cheek. *(N802.41)*

Fig. 327. Fracture of the zygoma showing flattening of the cheek and a fading circumorbital ecchymosis: x-ray **fig. 328.** *(N802.41)*

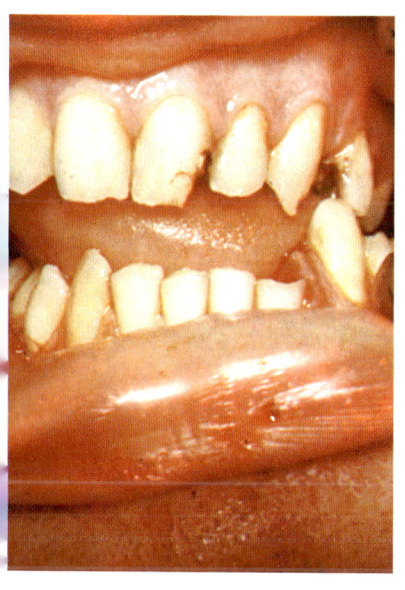
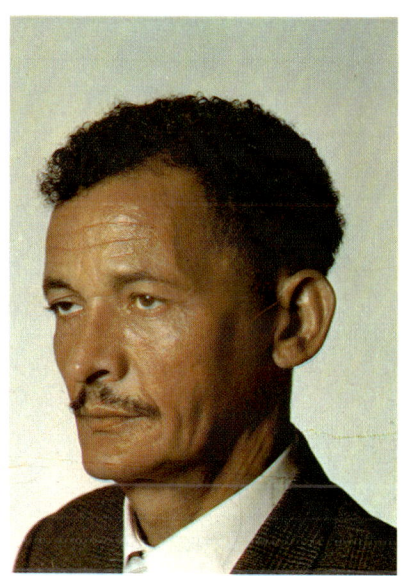
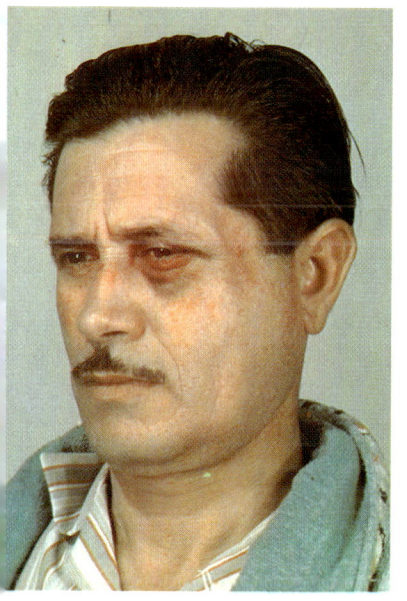
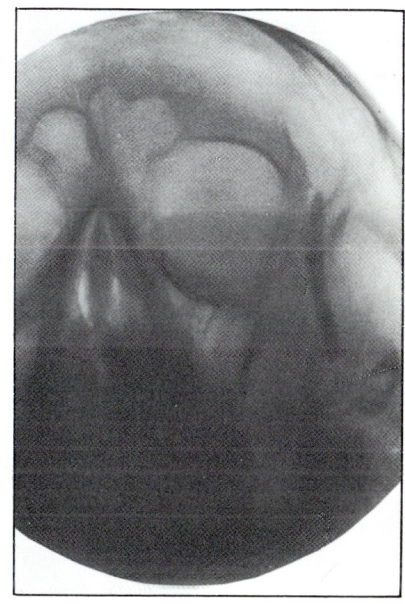

Index

[*References are to figure numbers, not page numbers*]

Abrasion, 76, 77
Abscess, 48, 49, 50, 51, 52, 53, 55, 56, 57, 58, 59, 60, 61, 62, 93
Actinic keratosis, 31
Actinomycosis, 48
Adenoma, 27, 159, 168, 180
Agranulocytosis, 123
Amelanotic melanoma, 153, 154
Amelogenesis imperfecta, 78, 79, 80, 81, 86
Anaesthesia (mental), 68, 220
Angiosarcoma, 155
Antibiotics, 5, 6, 71, 85, 201, 202
Anticoagulants, 8, 40
Antral
 carcinoma, 193, 194, 195, 196
 polyp, 137, 142, 150
Aphthous ulcer, 263, 265, 266, 268
Arsenic necrosis, 286
Aspirin burn, 247
Atrophy,
 mucosa, 207, 210
 tongue, 206

Basal cell carcinoma, 22
Betel-nut stain, 75
Bismuth, 122
Black hairy tongue, 201
Branchial,
 arch syndrome, 288, 289, 290, 291, 292, 293, 294, 295
 cyst, 66
Brown tongue, 202
Burkitt's lymphoma, 164
Burn,
 aspirin, 247
 thermal, 36

Calculus,
 dental, 109, 114
 submandibular gland, 43, 169, 170
Cancrum oris, 41
Candidosis, 259
Carbuncle, 39
Carcinoma,
 antral, 193, 194, 195, 196
 basal cell, 22
 lip, 34
 metastatic, 166
 oral, 149, 151, 152, 165, 167, 205, 261, 262
Caries, 104, 210
"Chronological" hypoplasia, 78

Cleft palate, 184
Condyle,
 hyperplasia, 296-299
 hypoplasia, 288-295, 307-310
 osteochondroma, 304-306
Connation, 88, 89
Cyst,
 branchial, 66
 dental, 143, 144, 223, 225, 227, 228, 229, 230
 "idiopathic bone", 226
 keratocyst, 140, 191
 mucosal, 139
 retention 224

Dentinogenesis imperfecta, 82, 84
Dento-alveolar abscess, 49, 50, 51, 52, 53, 59, 60, 61, 62, 67, 93
Denture,
 granuloma, 173
 trauma, 275
Dislocation, 321
Disproportion, 91

Ecchymosis, 29
Emphysema (surgical), 9
Eosinophilic granuloma, 231-234, 236
Epithelial inlay, 174
Erythema multiforme, 276, 278, 279

Facial nerve, 10
Fibro-epithelial polyp, 95, 133, 134
Fibroma, 138
Fibrous dysplasia, 162
Fluorosis, 74
Fracture, 322, 323, 324, 325, 326, 327

Gemination, 88, 89
Giant-cell granuloma, 129, 137
Gingiva, 108, 115, 124, 125
Gingivitis, 110, 111, 112, 113, 115, 116, 117, 118, 119
Granuloma (denture), 173

Haemangioma, 17, 18, 19, 20, 21, 30, 38, 211
Haematoma, 40
Hand, foot & mouth, 282
Herpes,
 simplex, 29, 32, 271, 272, 273
 zoster, 3, 10, 26
Histiocytosis X, 231, 232, 233, 234, 236
Hutchinson's teeth, 72
Hypercementosis, 105
Hyperparathyroidism, 237
Hyperplasia condylar, 296-299
Hyperthropy (masseter), 300
Hypoglossal nerve, 206

Hypoplasia,
  condylar, 288-291, 292-295, 307-310
  teeth, 72, 73, 78, 79, 80, 81, 86, 87

Internal resorption (pulp), 94
Iron deficiency, 207

Keratoacanthoma, 33
Keratosis,
  candidal, 259
  frictional, 248, 260
  idiopathic, 267
  naevoid, 246
  solar, 31
  syphilitic, 204

Lead, 122
Leucoplakia, 267
Leukaemia, 29, 123, 128
Lichen planus, 251, 281
Lupus vulgaris, 23
Lymphadenopathy, 42, 125, 154
Lymphangioma, 15, 16

Masseter-hyperthropy, 300
Melanoma,
  benign, 190
  malignant, 25, 153, 189
Mercury, 122
Metastatic carcinoma, 166
Mitral stenosis, 1
Mucous patch, 203
Muscles (masticatory), 301, 302

Naevus (epithelial), 246
Necrosis (arsenic), 286
Neurofibromatosis (von
  Recklinghausen), 3, 26, 212
Neutropenia, 123

Odontome, 243, 244, 245
Open-bite, 87, 311-314
Osteochondroma, 304-306
Osteogenesis imperfecta, 28
Osteogenic sarcoma, 220-222
Osteoma, 145, 146, 214
Osteomyelitis, 58, 68, 69, 70
Osteoradionecrosis, 161, 241, 242
Overcrowding, 91

Paget's disease of bone, 4, 13, 14
Palsy,
  facial, 10
  hypoglossal, 206
Papillary hyperplasia, 183
Papilloma, 35, 134
Pemphigus, 269, 270, 280, 283
Pericoronitis, 53, 54, 55

Periodontitis, 109, 114, 115, 122
Peutz-Jegher's syndrome, 37
Phlebolith, 21
Pink-spot, 94
Pleomorphic adenoma, 27, 159, 168, 180
Poliomyelitis, 302, 303
Polyp,
  antral, 136, 141, 150
  fibro-epithelial, 133, 134
  pulp, 95
Prognathism, 315-320

Ramsey-Hunt syndrome, 10
Resorption (idiopathic internal), 94
Retained teeth, 92
Reticulum cell sarcoma, 124, 125
Rickets, 87

Sarcoma, 124, 125, 155, 163, 164, 220-222
Sclera blue, 28
Sebaceous cyst, 24
Sequestrum, 58, 69
Sialolithiasis, 43, 169, 170
Sicca syndrome, 209, 210
Sinus, 59, 60, 61, 63, 67, 68, 70
Solitary bone cyst, 226
Stain, 71, 74, 75, 83, 97, 102, 103
Sturge-Weber syndrome, 17, 18
Submandibular swelling, 42-43
Submasseteric abscess, 56-58
Subperiosteal osteomyelitis, 58, 68, 69
Supernumerary (tooth), 90
Syphilis, 2, 72, 203, 204

Tetracycline staining, 71, 85
Torus mandibularis, 171
Torus palatinus, 179
Tuberculosis, 23

Ulcer,
  aphthous, 263, 265, 266, 268
  discoid lupus erythematosus, 277
  erythema multiforme, 276, 278, 279
  fusospirochaetal, 41, 116, 117, 118, 119,
                    123, 287
  lichen planus, 281
  neoplastic, 149, 151, 152, 155, 163, 165, 167,
              205
  neuropathic, 284
  traumatic, 156, 253, 274, 275
Uraemia, 257, 258

Vincent's infection, 116, 117, 118, 119,
                    123, 287
Von Recklinghausen's disease
  (neurofibromatosis), 3, 26, 212

Zoster (herpes), 3, 10, 26